Recent Advances in Geriatric Medicine

Volume 1

Chronic Diseases in Geriatric Patients

Tuck Yean Yong

Internal Medicine, Flinders Private Hospital

Flinders Drive, Bedford Park

South Australia 5042

Australia

Bentham Science Publishers Ltd.
Executive Suite Y - 2
PO Box 7917, Saif Zone
Sharjah, U.A.E.
Email: subscriptions@benthamscience.org

BENTHAM SCIENCE

CONTENTS

PREFACE

A rise in prevalence of chronic non-communicable diseases, including heart disease, hypertension, chronic obstructive pulmonary disease, chronic kidney disease, diabetes mellitus, stroke, cancers and osteoarthritis, have been observed among older people in many countries [1, 2]. A substantial and increased proportion of morbidity and mortality due to chronic disease occurs in older people. To compound this burden on the older individual and society in general, effective intervention is complicated by ageism, complex multiple comorbidity and lack of access to age-appropriate care. The purpose of this book is to address some of the medical care needs that exist for eleven common chronic conditions in older people. An additional chapter on end-of-life care will address the needs of older people with chronic diseases as they approach the terminal phase of life.

The chapter on coronary artery disease (CAD) in the elderly will look at the epidemiology, differences in clinical presentations and approach to evaluation and management that is appropriate for this age group. In particular issues on invasive assessment of the coronary artery and revascularisation procedures in older people with CAD will be addressed.

Heart failure is common in the older population and is associated with a poor prognosis. Managing older people with heart failure is a challenge because presenting features can be different from younger patients and the risk of adverse effects from polypharmacy. The chapter on heart failure aims to address these issues.

Hypertension is a common chronic condition in older people and an important risk factor for many vascular diseases. Therefore, the chapter on hypertension in older people will examine the evidence for controlling hypertension, target blood pressure and which antihypertensive agents to use in this age group.

Diabetes mellitus, especially type 2 diabetes, is a condition that affects many older people, about 20% of those aged ≥65 years. Like younger people, diabetes in the older age group is associated with significant morbidity, reduction in quality of life and mortality. In the older population, diabetes is associated with an increased risk of geriatric syndromes such as cognitive impairment, urinary incontinence and falls, which require careful assessment and management. The chapter on diabetes mellitus will look at some of the chronic problems faced by older people living with this condition.

Alzheimer's disease has emerged as a major public health concern globally which has a significant impact on the patient, family, caregivers and health care system. Although it has been recognised for more than a century, its pathogenesis is still not understood and benefits from pharmacological treatment has been limited so far. The chapter on Alzheimer's disease will provide updates on neuroimaging, nonpharmacological and pharmacological treatment.

Ischaemic stroke is associated with one of the highest causes of disability in older people. Evidence suggest that older people with ischaemic stroke often receive less effective therapy and experience poorer outcomes compared with younger patients. The chapter on ischaemic stroke in this book will review the available evidence on secondary prevention and treatment of this condition in older people and reducing the disability burden among survivors after the acute event.

Many older people have chronic obstructive pulmonary disease (COPD) as a result of smoking and age-related pulmonary changes. COPD is associated with increased morbidity and mortality for the older population. The chapter on COPD will look at the diagnostic and therapeutic aspects of this condition that are relevant to the older age group.

Cancers are increasingly diagnosed among people aged ≥65 years and this age group makes up more than 50% of new diagnosis of malignancy. Cancer care in older people is complex and challenging which is further compounded by limited evidence on the risk-benefit of treatments. The chapter on cancers in the elderly will review the differences in approach to management and identify gaps in evidence related to care of this group of older patients.

Osteoarthritis, especially in the hip or knee, is a common diagnosis in older people that causes significant pain leading to disability and decreased quality of life. Management of osteoarthritis in these joints among the elderly is challenging because they often have multiple chronic conditions that can compound pain and increased susceptibility to adverse effects of analgesics. The chapter on osteoarthritis will review evidence-based nonpharmacological, pharmacological and surgical approaches to management of this condition in the hips and knees of older people.

Osteoporosis and fragility fractures are highly prevalent in older people, with the latter associated with significant disability, mortality and health care cost. Osteoporosis is still underdiagnosed and undertreated among older people. The chapter on osteoporosis will examine the efficacy of both nonpharmacological and pharmacological strategies in the management of this condition and prevention of associated fragility fractures among the older population.

The prevalence of chronic kidney disease (CKD) in the older population is steadily increasing worldwide. Management of CKD in older people is complex because there are many competing factors that have to be taken into consideration. One of the chapters will attempt to untangle some of these complexities and provide an updated review on a holistic approach in management of older people with CKD.

As most of the chronic diseases described in this book have no cure, it is inevitable that these diseases will affect older people at the end of life. Evidence indicates that technology-driven interventions at the end of life do not necessarily improve satisfaction with care or quality of life. As a result, the final chapter of this book will address the need for advanced care planning and provision of good quality end-of-life care that is in concordance with the older patients' and their family's or caregivers' goals.

In this book, the authors have sought to provide educational and updated reviews on common chronic diseases encountered in geriatric medicine. Although the chapters in this book are not an exhaustive list of all chronic diseases, they review conditions that are frequently managed as part of day-to-day clinical practice. Managing older people with chronic diseases require a holistic approach with comprehensive assessment, leading to well integrated continuing care and focusing foremost on patients' goals in an effort to streamline care.

REFERENCES

[1] Freedman VA, Martin LG, Pell JP. Contribution of chronic conditions to aggregate changes in old-age functioning. Am J Public Health 2000; 90(11): 1755-60.
[PMID: PMC1446390]

[2] Bhattacharya J, Choudhry K, Lakdawalla D. Chronic disease and severe disability among working-age populations. Med Care 2005; 46(1): 92-100.
[PMID: 18162861]

Tuck Yean Yong
Internal Medicine, Flinders Private Hospital
Flinders Drive, Bedford Park
South Australia 5042
Australia

List of Contributors

Danielle Wu	Department of Nephrology, Mackay Base Hospital, Mackay, Australia
Kareeann Sok Fun Khow	Aged and Extended Care Services, The Queen Elizabeth Hospital and Department of Medicine, University of Adelaide, Adelaide, South Australia, Australia
Lei Gao	Department of Cardiology, General Hospital of People's Liberation Army, Beijing 100853, People's Republic of China
Tuck Yean Yong	Internal Medicine, Flinders Private Hospital, Flinders Drive, Bedford Park, Australia

Recent Advances in Geriatric Medicine

Recent Advances in Geriatric Medicine

Volume # 1

ISSN (Online): 2468-225X

ISSN: Print: 2468-2241

Chronic Diseases in Geriatric Patients

Editor: Tuck Yean Yong

ISBN (eBook): 978-1-68108-245-5

ISBN (Print): 978-1-68108-246-2

Reprints and Revisions:

First published in 2016

CHAPTER 1

Conundrums in the Care of Older Adults with Coronary Artery Disease

Lei Gao[*]

Department of Cardiology, General Hospital of People's Liberation Army, Beijing 100853, People's Republic of China

Abstract: Coronary artery disease (CAD) is one of the leading causes of death in both men and women aged > 65 years. However, older patients have been underrepresented in clinical trials resulting in limited data about the effectiveness of different treatment strategies in this population. Furthermore, the atypical clinical presentations of CAD in elderly patients, often make diagnosis challenging and can lead to suboptimal implementation of treatment and secondary preventive measures by health care professionals. This chapter reviews clinical presentations and diagnosis consideration of CAD in the elderly. This review will also address clinical challenges that often arise when considering medication therapy and percutaneous coronary intervention (PCI) in the elderly, as well as cardiac rehabilitation in this population. To optimize the benefits of therapy in the elderly, providers should consider complex interplay of variables such as comorbidities, functional and socioeconomic status, side effects associated with multiple drug administration, and individual biological variability.

Keywords: Acute coronary syndrome, Angina, Bleeding risk, Coronary artery disease, Medication therapy, Older adults, Percutaneous coronary intervention, Polypharmacy, Revascularization.

OVERVIEW OF CORONARY ARTERY DISEASE IN THE ELDERLY

The clinical manifestations of coronary artery disease (CAD) in older patients represent the effects of the disease superimposed on the physiological

[*] **Correspondence author Lei Gao:** Department of Cardiology, General Hospital of People's Liberation Army, Beijing 100853, People's Republic of China; Tel: +68 10 5549 9339; Fax: +68 10 5549 9339; E-mail: nkgaolei2010@126.com.

Tuck Yean Yong (Ed)

effects of age. Mortality and morbidity from CAD is strongly associated with increasing age. The age–sex standardized mortality rate for age <75 years is 56 per 100,000 population, compared with 1437 per 100,000 population among those aged ≥ 75 years [1]. Amongst people aged ≥ 75 years, more than one third of men and approximately one quarter of women have been observed to have CAD [1]. As a consequence of population aging, it is estimated that the total elderly population will rise by 42% over the next decade [2 - 7]. As a result, older people will account for an increasing proportion of patients using healthcare services for treatment of symptomatic CAD. Autopsy studies show that more than one half of people older than 60 years of age have significant CAD, with high prevalence of left main or triple-vessel disease [3]. Coronary angiography studies also showed old patients have more extensive and complicated coronary artery disease, more frequent multivessel disease, more calcification of coronary artery, and are more likely to have had previous myocardial infarction (MI) [8, 9].

CLINICAL PRESENTATION OF CORONARY ARTERY DISEASE IN THE ELDERLY

Although CAD is prevalent in elderly persons, the disease is often not diagnosed or misdiagnosed in this age group. Failure to correctly diagnose the disease in the elderly may be due to differences in the clinical manifestation in this age group compared with younger patients. Such differences may reflect a difference in the disease process between older and younger patients or it may be related to the superimposition of normal aging changes. In addition, the presence of concomitant diseases may mask the usual clinical manifestations. An increased proportion of older patients compared to younger ones have atypical manifestations of myocardial ischemia, including dyspnoea and worsening heart failure [10]. Additionally, the frequent coexistence of chronic lung disease, gastroesophageal reflux disease, and other disorders may make CAD diagnosis more challenging. On the other hand, reductions in physical activity and aerobic exercise capacity may mask the symptoms in elderly CAD patients. The frequent coexistence of chronic lung disease, peripheral vascular disease, arthritis, and neurological disorders may make ambulation difficult. Therefore, a lack of exertional angina in an elderly patient with suspected CHD may merely reflect the patient's lack of significant activity. Clinical manifestation of acute coronary syndrome (ACS) in the elderly may be more complicated [11]. Atypical presentations, absence of chest pain, dyspnoea, and symptoms related to comorbid diseases are common in elderly with ACS. Electrocardiographic changes are more often equivocal in the elderly, because of pre-existing bundle branch block or residual ST-elevation from previous infarct wall, and make electrocardiographic interpretation challenging. Cardiac troponin elevation can be seen in conditions other than ST-segment elevation myocardial infarction (STEMI), and many of these conditions such as heart failure, pulmonary embolism, sepsis, end-stage kidney disease, stroke, and so on are increasingly prevalent with age [12].

DIAGNOSTIC CONSIDERATION OF CAD IN THE ELDERLY

The evaluation of an older person with suspected CAD should begin with a detailed history and full physical examination, and ascertainment of the coronary risk factors and comorbid illnesses. After initial assessment of clinical stability, it is necessary to stratify patients to high- or low-risk group. Clinical outcomes in elderly patients with CAD are directly related to left ventricular function, the extent of vascular disease, and the presence of comorbidities [9, 10]. So assessment of heart function and coronary artery lesion severity by noninvasive or invasive imaging tests are also important. Additionally, stress testing is critical in stratifying older patients with myocardial ischemia, especially those who are asymptomatic.

SPECIAL CONSIDERATIONS FOR MEDICAL THERAPY IN ELDERLY PATIENTS WITH CAD

The principal goals in the care of patients with CAD, are to establish the diagnosis, relieve symptoms, and to prevent future cardiac events such as ACS, revascularization, or death. Pharmacological therapy plays an important role in achieving these goals. Beta (β)-blockers are preferred for initial treatment of symptoms. Calcium channel blockers and nitrates can be used to provide symptom relief when initial treatment with β-blockers is ineffective, contraindicated or causing side effects. Ranolazine, a piperazine derivative, produces its antianginal effects without decreasing heart rate or blood pressure. Ranolazine has been used effective in improving angina symptom in patients who did respond to nitrates, β-blockers, or calcium channel blockers [13]. Additionally, therapies known to reduce the incidence of adverse cardiovascular events such as death and myocardial infarction should be also be started when the patents are diagnosed CAD. These include aspirin, statin, smoking cessation, control of blood pressure and excess weight, and optimal management of diabetes. In the recent guidelines for the management of CAD, medications such as aspirin, β-blockers, calcium channel blockers, statins, nitrates, anticoagulants, and antiplatelet agents were found to be as effective and safe in the older population [14, 15]. Aspirin should be maintained at 81 mg per day for older patients after stent insertion. Due to the risk of excessive bleeding without clinical benefit, the U.S. Food and Drug Administration listed a Black Box warning that does not recommend administration of prasugrel in patients with ACS who are ≥75 years of age or weigh <60 kg except for those at very high risk [16].

Considerations should be given to potential adverse effects of pharmacological treatment in the elderly patient with CAD. Marked vasodilation resulting from rapid absorption or higher peak effects of isosorbide dinitrates can cause postural hypotension. Therefore, agents with smoother concentration *versus* time profiles such as mononitrates or transdermal formulations are preferred. β-blockers have not been shown to increase the occurrence of depression in previous studies, but agents that are not lipophilic (*e.g.*, atenolol, nadolol) may produce fewer central nervous system effects [17]. Additionally, calcium channel blockers, especially the dihydropyridines, have a tendency to cause pedal edema more frequently in the older patient. Shorter acting formulations can cause or worsen postural hypotension and should be avoided in older people prone to falls. Verapamil can exacerbate constipation, especially in older people who are sedentary.

Given that multiple comorbidities are common in the elderly, the rate of polypharmacy with use of 5 or more drugs is high in this population. With the increased number of concurrent medications and potential for drug-drug interactions, risk of adverse effects is an important consideration for older patients with CAD. In one analysis of 750 nursing home residents with mean age of 85 years (range 65–108), Beloosesky *et al.* found 42.6% of residents were taking more than 5 drugs [18]. Many older adults with CAD have multiple medical conditions that require medical attention, exposing them to polypharmacy and a higher risk of being prescribed potentially inappropriate medications. These situations may cause adverse drug reactions, longer hospital stays, and death. In a cross-sectional survey of a community dwelling population aged 60 years and older, the prevalence of polypharmacy with use of four or more medications was close to 30% [19].

Whenever possible, primary care physicians should use evidence-based non-pharmacological interventions that are appropriate. In addition, better understanding of aging-related physiology and pharmacology can help to minimize iatrogenic complications of commonly used drugs in this vulnerable population. Therefore, current treatment guidelines should be adopted cautiously in elderly patients, particularly those older than 75 years, with careful assessment of concurrent medications and consideration of initiating specific drugs such as statin at lower doses [20]. Advanced age, female sex, small body size, fatty liver disease, and multisystem disease may predispose to adverse events associated with statin use. In addition, lipophilic statins such as lovastatin, simvastatin, and atorvastatin, are metabolized *via* the cytochrome P450 system, predisposing to interactions with other drugs metabolized by this pathway [21].

REVASCULARIZATION FOR OLDER PATIENTS WITH CAD

Revascularization procedures among elderly patients are increasingly common. In current practice, more than 1 in 5 patients treated with percutaneous coronary intervention (PCI) are aged ≥75 years and the proportion of older individuals in this treatment group is growing [9]. Older patients have more cardiovascular risk factors and a greater burden of disease compared with younger patients needing revascularization and, therefore, are more likely to derive greater benefit from revascularization. However, they are also more likely to experience procedure-related complications, because of age-related physiological changes, frailty, and comorbidities [9]. PCI is associated with a slightly <1% risk of stroke or coma, and coronary artery bypass grafting (CABG) is associated with a 3-6% incidence of permanent stroke or coma in patients aged >75 years [22]. Early CABG mortality increased from <2% in patients younger than 60 years of age to 6-8% in octogenarians in recent series [23]. Registry data also show that mortality risk for PCI increases with age from approximately 1% for those less than 70 years of age, to approximately 2% for those aged 70-80 years, and 3.2% for those older than 80 years [24]. Post-PCI bleeding and acute kidney injury are more common in the elderly population and are associated with high readmission rate [9].

Therefore, the decision on when to pursue revascularization in elderly patients, and if so, how to revascularize, is relatively complicated. To optimize the benefits of revascularization therapy in older people, patients and their care providers need to have an informed discussion about objectives of treatment and related risks of PCI or CABG and alternative therapies. Once a decision to undergo PCI or CABG is reached, clinicians need to address modifiable risks for complications such as bleeding, stroke, acute kidney injury. Clinicians also need to individualize care decisions, and pay careful attention to treatment selection (such as choice of adjuvant therapies and timing of revascularization) and drug dosage. For many elderly patients, the net benefits of revascularization with PCI or CABG regarding whether symptom control, quality of life (QoL), morbidity and mortality may surpass the associated risks [9].

Approach to choosing between CABG and PCI in the elderly patients is another complex problem. Classically, CABG has been considered the most effective revascularization approach, and in the past, certain clinical findings have been regarded as "absolute" indications for a surgical intervention. Multivessel disease, left main disease and the presence of multiple, and severely calcified lesions are indications for CABG. A recent comprehensive analysis linked data from the ACC and the STS Adult Cardiac Surgery database with claims data from Centers for Medicare and Medicaid Services to analyze outcomes with CABG and PCI in U.S. patients 65 years of age or older with multivessel disease without acute myocardial infarction. The data confirmed trends of earlier randomized studies showing no difference in adjusted mortality between the CABG *versus* PCI groups at one year after the procedure and a lower mortality with CABG than with PCI at four years [24]. However, recently PCI has been demonstrated to be increasingly effective, even in cases which were previously absolute indications for surgery. Drug-eluting stents, intravascular imaging modalities, fractional-flow reserve measurements and rotational atherectomy devices are among the new technology that has increased PCI efficacy and application [25]. Whether these new techniques will safely extend the reach of PCI to obviate the need for surgery is the subject of intensive research.

CARDIAC REHABILITATION FOR OLDER PEOPLE WITH CAD

Components of secondary prevention programming (including exercise; smoking cessation; management of dyslipidemia, hypertension, diabetes, and weight; and interventions directed at depression, social isolation, return to work, and other psychosocial issues) can be provided by the clinician in the office setting or through cardiac rehabilitation programs. Cardiac rehabilitation programs are particularly well suited to the implementation of secondary prevention services. However, many older patients who would derive benefit from these interventions unfortunately do not participate because of a lack of referral or societal and other barriers [26].

ADDITIONAL CONSIDERATIONS FOR REVASCULARIZATION IN THE ELDERLY: BLEEDING RISKS AND ACUTE KIDNEY INJURY

Bleeding and transfusion rates are higher in older patients, especially with improper dosing of anticoagulation, antiplatelet and antithrombin agents, glycoprotein (GP) IIb/IIIa inhibitors, and dual antiplatelet therapy. Those at high risk for intracerebral hemorrhage include patients older than 75 years, women, African Americans, smaller patients (<65 kg in women and <80 kg for men), previous stroke, and systolic blood pressure greater than 160 mmHg [27]. Bleeding risk including intracerebral haemorrhage is increased by approximately two-fold with GP IIb/IIIa inhibitors, rising to 7.2% for eptifibatide in patients older than 80 years of age [28]. The CathPCI Registry study evaluated trends in use of bleeding avoidance strategies (direct thrombin inhibitors, vascular closure devices, and radial access) and risk-adjusted bleeding over time [29]. Of 10,469 patients aged >80 years undergoing primary PCI, 1,002 (9.6%) developed a bleeding complication. In multivariable analysis, use of bleeding avoidance strategies was associated with a lower risk of bleeding.

Recent studies showed that transradial primary percutaneous intervention, particularly by preventing access site bleeding, was associated with a significantly lower mortality compared with the femoral approach [30]. The RIVAL (Radial *versus* femoral access for coronary angiography and intervention in patients with acute coronary syndromes) investigators reported a significantly lower rate of vascular complications in their randomized, parallel-group, multicenter study of patients undergoing PCI for STEMI, resulting in a reduction in overall mortality in the radial access group [31]. The transradial approach may also increase the success rate of primary PCI in the elderly by circumventing the procedural problems related to peripheral artery disease, and may overcome the difficulty in passing through tortuous femoral, iliac, abdominal, and thoracic aortae. However, older age is a risk for radial access failure that is related as well to operator experience [32]. Experience with the radial approach in the U.S currently lags that of Asia and Europe [33].

In addition, antithrombotic treatment should also be tailored in patients over 80 years of age to prevent major bleeding complications. A direct thrombin inhibitor, bivalirudin, has gained a Class Ib recommendation as a supportive measure for primary PCI [34]. A prespecified age subgroup analysis of the ACUITY (Acute Catheterization and Urgent Intervention Triage Strategy) study has recently demonstrated that although there were no significant differences in efficacy, the benefit of bivalirudin in terms of absolute reduction in bleeding events is most pronounced in patients > 75 years of age [35].

Relative benefit and harm of GP IIb/IIIa inhibitor use varies across age strata. Compared with younger patients, GP IIb/IIIa inhibitor was observed to have a lower efficacy and disproportionate rates of bleeding in older patients. These unfavorable outcomes may be improved by careful patient selection and GP IIb/IIIa inhibitor avoidance in patients who do not require PCI. Notably, estimation of creatinine clearance and weight are strictly recommended to avoid overdosing, particularly in the elderly. Dose adjustment is recommended for eptifibatide and tirofiban in patients with reduced renal function. Additionally, in elderly patients receiving GP IIb/IIIa inhibitors, the number of antithrombotic drugs used should be balanced against the individual risk of thrombotic and bleeding complications. Overall, the presently established strategies to prevent major bleeding in octogenarians include very careful usage of glycoprotein IIb/IIIa inhibitors, considering use of bivalirudin for primary PCI, considering low-dose aspirin (81 mg) for chronic antiplatelet therapy, and avoiding triple anticoagulant therapy (aspirin, clopidogrel, warfarin) when possible [36].

Potential strategies include adjusting doses of aspirin and clopidogrel based upon point-of-care platelet function assays and selecting the radial artery routinely for arterial access.

Acute kidney injury is another important complication of revascularization in the older patients with STEMI. It is known to be associated with both urgent coronary angiography and advanced age. Fig. (**1**) shows predictors of contrast induced acute kidney injury [37]. The volume of contrast medium used during urgent coronary intervention tends to be relatively higher than in elective procedures. Accordingly, adequate hydration before and after exposure to contrast medium, along with avoidance of nephrotoxic drugs, remains the recommended prophylaxis against acute kidney injury [38]. Recent clinical evidence does not support the use of N-acetylcysteine for prophylaxis against acute kidney injury [39, 40].

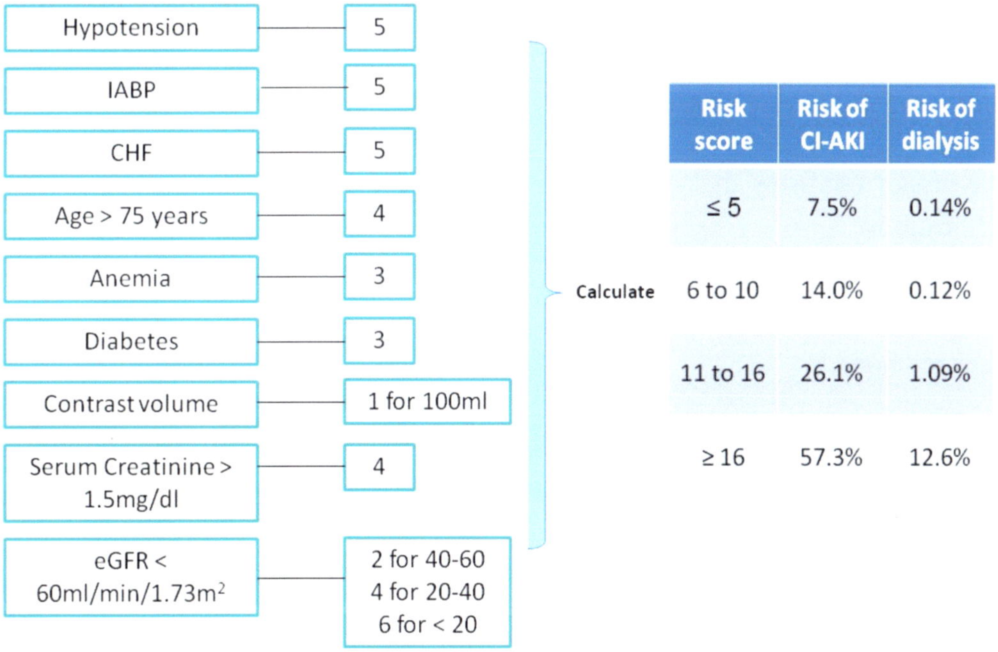

Fig. (1). Risk score to assess contrast-induced acute kidney injury (CI-AKI).

CONCLUSION

The changing demographics of heart disease has sharpened the focus on optimization of therapy in the older people with CAD. Age-associated pathophysiological changes make the elderly a high-risk group in terms of mortality and adverse events in the setting of CAD, especially when ACS occurs. However, given their high-risk status, the elderly with CAD are also a group that is very likely to experience improvements in clinical outcomes and functional status with the use of pharmacological and revascularization therapy. As such, the decision on when to pursue revascularization in older patients, and if so, how to revascularize, is an important but complex one. For the purpose of achieving maximal benefits of treatment in the elderly with CAD, therapy should be individualized with therapeutic choices considering medical and cognitive status, anticipated life expectancy, and patient or family preferences and with early invasive strategies directed to the high-risk group who is more likely to derive the greatest benefit. Narrowing of current gaps in our knowledge in conjunction with advances in revascularization techniques and pharmacological options will enable improvement in outcomes and the appropriate selection of older people who are suitable to be treated with revascularization therapy.

CONFLICT OF INTEREST

The author confirms that author has no conflict of interest to declare for this publication.

ACKNOWLEDGEMENTS

Declared none.

KEY POINTS

- Clinical manifestations of coronary artery disease (CAD) in older adults are different from younger patients.
- Careful consideration with medical therapy to avoid polypharmacy and drug interactions in the elderly patient with CAD.
- Outcomes of revascularization procedures such as percutaneous coronary intervention or coronary artery bypass grafting for older patients with CAD will depend on appropriate selection.

REFERENCES

[1] Johnman C, Oldroyd KG, Pell JP. Elective percutaneous coronary intervention in the elderly patient. Aging Health 2011; 7: 271-81.
[http://dx.doi.org/10.2217/ahe.11.13]

[2] Alexander KP, Roe MT, Chen AY, *et al.* Evolution in cardiovascular care for elderly patients with non-ST-segment elevation acute coronary syndromes: results from the CRUSADE National Quality Improvement Initiative. J Am Coll Cardiol 2005; 46(8): 1479-87.
[http://dx.doi.org/10.1016/j.jacc.2005.05.084] [PMID: 16226171]

[3] Mehta RH, Rathore SS, Radford MJ, Wang Y, Wang Y, Krumholz HM. Acute myocardial infarction in the elderly: differences by age. J Am Coll Cardiol 2001; 38(3): 736-41.
[http://dx.doi.org/10.1016/S0735-1097(01)01432-2] [PMID: 11527626]

[4] From AM, Rihal CS, Lennon RJ, Holmes DR Jr, Prasad A. Temporal trends and improved outcomes of percutaneous coronary revascularization in nonagenarians. JACC Cardiovasc Interv 2008; 1(6): 692-8.
[http://dx.doi.org/10.1016/j.jcin.2008.07.009] [PMID: 19463386]

[5] Singh M, Peterson ED, Roe MT, *et al.* Trends in the association between age and in-hospital mortality after percutaneous coronary intervention: National Cardiovascular Data Registry experience. Circ Cardiovasc Interv 2009; 2(1): 20-6.
[http://dx.doi.org/10.1161/CIRCINTERVENTIONS.108.826172] [PMID: 20031689]

[6] Bauer T, Möllmann H, Weidinger F, *et al.* Predictors of hospital mortality in the elderly undergoing percutaneous coronary intervention for acute coronary syndromes and stable angina. Int J Cardiol 2011; 151(2): 164-9.
[http://dx.doi.org/10.1016/j.ijcard.2010.05.006] [PMID: 20605241]

[7] Steinman MA, Lee SJ, John Boscardin W, *et al.* Patterns of multimorbidity in elderly veterans. J Am Geriatr Soc 2012; 60(10): 1872-80.
[http://dx.doi.org/10.1111/j.1532-5415.2012.04158.x] [PMID: 23035702]

[8] Sugiura M, Hiraoka K, Ohkawa S. Severity of coronary sclerosis in the aged: a pathological study in 968 consecutive autopsy cases. Jpn Heart J 1976; 17(4): 471-8.
[http://dx.doi.org/10.1536/ihj.17.471] [PMID: 966383]

[9] Wang TY, Gutierrez A, Peterson ED. Percutaneous coronary intervention in the elderly. Nat Rev Cardiol 2011; 8(2): 79-90.
[http://dx.doi.org/10.1038/nrcardio.2010.184] [PMID: 21139558]

[10] Williams MA, Fleg JL, Ades PA, *et al.* Secondary prevention of coronary heart disease in the elderly (with emphasis on patients > or =75 years of age): an American heart association scientific statement from the council on clinical cardiology subcommittee on exercise, cardiac rehabilitation, and prevention. Circulation 2002; 105(14): 1735-43.
[http://dx.doi.org/10.1161/01.CIR.0000013074.73995.6C] [PMID: 11940556]

[11] Dangas GD, Singh HS. Primary percutaneous coronary intervention in octogenarians: navigate with caution. Heart 2010; 96(11): 813-4.
[http://dx.doi.org/10.1136/hrt.2009.191916] [PMID: 20478859]

[12] Inbar R, Shoenfeld Y. Elevated cardiac troponins: the ultimate marker for myocardial necrosis, but not without a differential diagnosis. Isr Med Assoc J 2009; 11(1): 50-3. [PMID: 19344014]

[13] Banon D, Filion KB, Budlovsky T, Franck C, Eisenberg MJ. The usefulness of ranolazine for the treatment of refractory chronic stable angina pectoris as determined from a systematic review of randomized controlled trials. Am J Cardiol 2014; 113(6): 1075-82. [http://dx.doi.org/10.1016/j.amjcard.2013.11.070] [PMID: 24462341]

[14] Antman EM, Hand M, Armstrong PW, *et al.* 2007 focused update of the ACC/AHA 2004 guidelines for the management of patients with ST-Elevation myocardial infarction: a report of the American college of cardiology/American heart association task force on practice guidelines: developed in collaboration with the Canadian cardiovascular society endorsed by the American academy of family physicians: 2007 writing group to review new evidence and update the ACC/AHA 2004 guidelines for the management of patients with ST-Elevation myocardial infarction, writing on behalf of the 2004 writing committee. Circulation 2008; 117(2): 296-329. [http://dx.doi.org/10.1161/CIRCULATIONAHA.107.188209] [PMID: 18071078]

[15] Anderson JL, Adams CD, Antman EM, *et al.* ACC/AHA 2007 guidelines for the management of patients with unstable angina/non-ST-Elevation myocardial infarction: a report of the American College of Cardiology/American Heart Association Task Force on Practice Guidelines (Writing Committee to Revise the 2002 Guidelines for the Management of Patients With Unstable Angina/Non-ST-Elevation Myocardial Infarction) developed in collaboration with the American College of Emergency Physicians, the Society for Cardiovascular Angiography and Interventions, and the Society of Thoracic Surgeons endorsed by the American Association of Cardiovascular and Pulmonary Rehabilitation and the Society for Academic Emergency Medicine. J Am Coll Cardiol 2007; 50(7): e1-e157. [http://dx.doi.org/10.1016/j.jacc.2007.02.013] [PMID: 17692738]

[16] Amsterdam EA, Wenger NK, Brindis RG, *et al.* 2014 AHA/ACC guideline for the management of patients with non-ST-Elevation acute coronary syndromes: a report of the American college of cardiology/American heart association task force on practice guidelines. J Am Coll Cardiol 2014; 64(24): e139-228. [http://dx.doi.org/10.1016/j.jacc.2014.09.017] [PMID: 25260718]

[17] Schwartz JB, Zipes DP. Cardiovascular disease in the elderly. In: Mann DL, Zipes DP, Libby P, Bonow RO, Eds. Braunwald's heart disease: A textbook of cardiovascular medicine. 10th ed. Philadelphia, PA: WB Saunders 2015; pp. 1711-43.

[18] Beloosesky Y, Nenaydenko O, Gross Nevo RF, Adunsky A, Weiss A. Rates, variability, and associated factors of polypharmacy in nursing home patients. Clin Interv Aging 2013; 8: 1585-90. [http://dx.doi.org/10.2147/CIA.S52698] [PMID: 24348028]

[19] Husson N, Watfa G, Laurain MC, *et al.* Characteristics of polymedicated ($\geq$ 4) elderly: a survey in a community-dwelling population aged 60 years and over. J Nutr Health Aging 2014; 18(1): 87-91. [http://dx.doi.org/10.1007/s12603-013-0337-8] [PMID: 24402395]

[20] Reiner Z, Catapano AL, De Backer G, *et al.* ESC/EAS Guidelines for the management of dyslipidaemias: the Task Force for the management of dyslipidaemias of the European Society of Cardiology (ESC) and the European Atherosclerosis Society (EAS). Eur Heart J 2011; 32(14): 1769-

818.
[http://dx.doi.org/10.1093/eurheartj/ehr158] [PMID: 21712404]

[21] Roberts CG, Guallar E, Rodriguez A. Efficacy and safety of statin monotherapy in older adults: a meta-analysis. J Gerontol A Biol Sci Med Sci 2007; 62(8): 879-87.
[http://dx.doi.org/10.1093/gerona/62.8.879] [PMID: 17702880]

[22] King SB III, Smith SC Jr, Hirshfeld JW Jr, *et al.* 2007 focused update of the ACC/AHA/SCAI 2005 guideline update for percutaneous coronary intervention: a report of the American College of Cardiology/American Heart Association Task Force on Practice guidelines. J Am Coll Cardiol 2008; 51(2): 172-209.
[http://dx.doi.org/10.1016/j.jacc.2007.10.002] [PMID: 18191745]

[23] Kurlansky P. Do octogenarians benefit from coronary artery bypass surgery: a question with a rapidly changing answer? Curr Opin Cardiol 2012; 27(6): 611-9.
[http://dx.doi.org/10.1097/HCO.0b013e328358b072] [PMID: 23037830]

[24] Singh M, Peterson ED, Milford-Beland S, Rumsfeld JS, Spertus JA. Validation of the Mayo clinic risk score for in-hospital mortality after percutaneous coronary interventions using the national cardiovascular data registry. Circ Cardiovasc Interv 2008; 1(1): 36-44.
[http://dx.doi.org/10.1161/CIRCINTERVENTIONS.107.755991] [PMID: 20031653]

[25] Levine GN, Bates ER, Blankenship JC, *et al.* 2011 ACCF/AHA/SCAI guideline for percutaneous coronary intervention. A report of the American college of cardiology foundation/American heart association task force on practice guidelines and the society for cardiovascular angiography and interventions. J Am Coll Cardiol 2011; 58(24): e44-e122.
[http://dx.doi.org/10.1016/j.jacc.2011.08.007] [PMID: 22070834]

[26] Ades PA, Waldmann ML, McCann WJ, Weaver SO. Predictors of cardiac rehabilitation participation in older coronary patients. Arch Intern Med 1992; 152(5): 1033-5.
[http://dx.doi.org/10.1001/archinte.1992.00400170113021] [PMID: 1580707]

[27] Weintraub WS, Grau-Sepulveda MV, Weiss JM, *et al.* Comparative effectiveness of revascularization strategies. N Engl J Med 2012; 366(16): 1467-76.
[http://dx.doi.org/10.1056/NEJMoa1110717] [PMID: 22452338]

[28] Alexander KP, Newby LK, Cannon CP, *et al.* Acute coronary care in the elderly, part I: Non-S--segment-elevation acute coronary syndromes: a scientific statement for healthcare professionals from the American Heart Association Council on Clinical Cardiology: in collaboration with the Society of Geriatric Cardiology. Circulation 2007; 115(19): 2549-69.
[http://dx.doi.org/10.1161/CIRCULATIONAHA.107.182615] [PMID: 17502590]

[29] Dodson JA, Wang Y, Chaudhry SI, Curtis JP. Bleeding-avoidance strategies and outcomes in patients ≥80 years of age with ST-elevation myocardial infarction undergoing primary percutaneous coronary intervention (from the NCDR CathPCI Registry). Am J Cardiol 2012; 110(1): 1-6.
[http://dx.doi.org/10.1016/j.amjcard.2012.02.039] [PMID: 22475362]

[30] Arzamendi D, Ly HQ, Tanguay JF, *et al.* Effect on bleeding, time to revascularization, and one-year clinical outcomes of the radial approach during primary percutaneous coronary intervention in patients with ST-segment elevation myocardial infarction. Am J Cardiol 2010; 106(2): 148-54.
[http://dx.doi.org/10.1016/j.amjcard.2010.02.028] [PMID: 20598995]

[31] Jolly SS, Yusuf S, Cairns J, *et al.* Radial *versus* femoral access for coronary angiography and intervention in patients with acute coronary syndromes (RIVAL): a randomised, parallel group, multicentre trial. Lancet 2011; 377(9775): 1409-20.
[http://dx.doi.org/10.1016/S0140-6736(11)60404-2] [PMID: 21470671]

[32] Khan R, Ly HQ. Transradial percutaneous coronary interventions in acute coronary syndrome. Am J Cardiol 2014; 114(1): 160-8.
[http://dx.doi.org/10.1016/j.amjcard.2014.04.017] [PMID: 24925803]

[33] Rao SV, Dai D, Subherwal S, *et al.* Association between periprocedural bleeding and long-term outcomes following percutaneous coronary intervention in older patients. JACC Cardiovasc Interv 2012; 5(9): 958-65.
[http://dx.doi.org/10.1016/j.jcin.2012.05.010] [PMID: 22995883]

[34] O'Gara PT, Kushner FG, Ascheim DD, *et al.* 2013 ACCF/AHA guideline for the management of ST-elevation myocardial infarction: a report of the American College of Cardiology Foundation/American Heart Association Task Force on Practice Guidelines. J Am Coll Cardiol 2013; 61(4): e78-e140.
[http://dx.doi.org/10.1016/j.jacc.2012.11.019] [PMID: 23256914]

[35] Lopes RD, Alexander KP, Manoukian SV, *et al.* Advanced age, antithrombotic strategy, and bleeding in non-ST-segment elevation acute coronary syndromes: results from the ACUITY (Acute Catheterization and Urgent Intervention Triage Strategy) trial. J Am Coll Cardiol 2009; 53(12): 1021-30.
[http://dx.doi.org/10.1016/j.jacc.2008.12.021] [PMID: 19298914]

[36] Capodanno D, Angiolillo DJ. Antithrombotic therapy in the elderly. J Am Coll Cardiol 2010; 56(21): 1683-92.
[http://dx.doi.org/10.1016/j.jacc.2010.04.063] [PMID: 21070918]

[37] Mehran R, Aymong ED, Nikolsky E, *et al.* A simple risk score for prediction of contrast-induced nephropathy after percutaneous coronary intervention: development and initial validation. J Am Coll Cardiol 2004; 44(7): 1393-9.
[PMID: 15464318]

[38] Sadat U. N-acetylcysteine in contrast-induced acute kidney injury: clinical use against principles of evidence-based clinical medicine! Expert Rev Cardiovasc Ther 2014; 12(1): 1-3.
[http://dx.doi.org/10.1586/14779072.2014.852066] [PMID: 24236859]

[39] Investigators AC. Acetylcysteine for prevention of renal outcomes in patients undergoing coronary and peripheral vascular angiography: main results from the randomized Acetylcysteine for Contrast-induced nephropathy Trial (ACT). Circulation 2011; 124(11): 1250-9.
[http://dx.doi.org/10.1161/CIRCULATIONAHA.111.038943] [PMID: 21859972]

[40] Erturk M, Uslu N, Gorgulu S, *et al.* Does intravenous or oral high-dose N-acetylcysteine in addition to saline prevent contrast-induced nephropathy assessed by cystatin C? Coron Artery Dis 2014; 25(2): 111-7.
[http://dx.doi.org/10.1097/MCA.0000000000000073] [PMID: 24365793]

CHAPTER 2

Treating the "Young at Heart": Management of Heart Failure in the Older Population

Tuck Yean Yong[1,*], **Kareeann Sok Fun Khow**[2]

[1] *Internal Medicine, Flinders Private Hospital, Flinders Drive, Bedford Park, South Australia 5042, Australia*

[2] *Aged and Extended Care Services, The Queen Elizabeth Hospital and Department of Medicine, University of Adelaide, Adelaide, South Australia, Australia*

Abstract: The prevalence of heart failure rises with increasing age. Although patients with heart failure are mainly elderly (age ≥65 years), evidence for efficacious diagnostic and therapeutic approaches are limited in this population. Diagnosis of heart failure in older people is challenging because of comorbidities masking symptoms and signs; different diagnostic cut-offs of natriuretic peptides; and the high prevalence of heart failure with preserved ejection fraction (HFPEF). Geriatric syndromes (such as cognitive impairment, frailty, falls and incontinence) are common in heart failure and can affect patients' prognosis. In older patients with reduced ejection fraction, angiotensin-converting enzyme inhibitors, angiotensin receptor blockers and beta-blockers have improved clinical outcomes. However no therapeutic strategy has yet been found to improve prognosis of HFPEF which affect many older people.

Keywords: Ageing, Cardiac devices, Diagnosis, Ejection fraction, Elderly, Geriatric syndromes, Heart failure, Left ventricular function, Systolic dysfunction, Therapy.

INTRODUCTION

Heart failure is largely a disorder of the older people and as the population ages; its prevalence is expected to rise to epidemic proportion [1]. People aged 65 years

* **Correspondence author Tuck Yean Yong:** Internal Medicine, Flinders Private Hospital, Flinders Drive, Bedford Park, South Australia 5042, Australia; Tel: +61 8 8241 2121; Fax: 8240 0879; E-mail: tyyong@hotmail.com.

and older account for more than 75% of hospitalizations related to heart failure [2]. In the US each year, nearly ten new cases of heart failure are diagnosed in every 1000 people aged over 65 years [3]. The American College of Cardiology and American Heart Association defines heart failure as "a complex clinical syndrome that can result from any structural or functional cardiac disorder that impairs the ability of the ventricle to fill with or eject blood" [3].

Although heart failure occurs more frequently in older people, current diagnostic and therapeutic recommendations are derived largely from studies that have included few people in this age group. The purpose of this chapter is to review the diagnosis of heart failure in older people and effectiveness of different management strategies including non-pharmacological, pharmacological, common associated geriatric syndromes and device-related therapies in this age group.

CLINICAL FEATURES

Fatigue or dyspnoea on exertion, with or without some degree of peripheral oedema, are the more common early symptoms of heart failure in older people [4]. With progression of heart failure, especially if untreated, dyspnea on exertion eventually occurs even at rest or fatigue becomes more severe. Such symptom may not always be apparent in older people because of restricted physical activities, therefore delaying diagnosis. Orthopnoea and paroxysmal nocturnal dyspnea are more specific symptoms for heart failure in older people [4, 5]. Oedema associated with heart failure is always symmetrical and pitting. It generally begins with foot and ankle, extends proximally and can involve the scrotal area, sacral region and abdomen. Chronic severe oedema can lead to skin changes such as brown pigmentation, induration and skin blisters. Other less frequent and atypical symptoms of heart failure in older people include syncope, angina, nocturia, oliguria and changes in mental status.

In the physical examination of an older person with heart failure, an elevated jugular venous pressure is the most specific sign of fluid overload [6]. Other physical signs such as pulmonary crackles, third heart sound or leg oedema may not always be present in chronic heart failure and may be caused by other conditions [7].

EVALUATION OF HEART FAILURE IN OLDER PATIENTS

Heart failure has to be evaluated as a syndrome and not a disease. It often has an identifiable underlying cause. Coronary artery disease and hypertension are two of the more common causes of heart failure across all age groups, including older people [8, 9].

The most clinically relevant classification of heart failure into systolic dysfunction or preserved systolic function is based on left ventricular ejection fraction, which is most commonly assessed by transthoracic echocardiography. Determining if the systolic function is preserved or not has both prognostic and therapeutic implications [10]. Heart failure with reduced left ventricular ejection fraction is defined as clinical heart failure with left ventricular ejection fraction <45% [11]. Systolic heart failure is characterized by an enlarged and weakened left ventricle that is impaired in producing a normal stroke volume and cardiac output. Epidemiological data suggest that about 50% of all heart failure patients have a preserved ejection fraction, also known as diastolic heart failure [12]. Heart failure with preserved left ventricular ejection fraction (HFPEF) is defined as clinical heart failure with normal or near normal left ventricular ejection fraction, generally 55% or greater [13]. To make a clinical diagnosis of HFPEF, determination of diastolic dysfunction is not essential but abnormalities in active and passive relaxation are commonly observed [14]. Over half of all heart failure in the older population have normal left ventricular ejection fraction [15].

Measuring plasma levels of brain natriuretic peptide (BNP) is useful for the triage of patients with suspected heart failure [16]. BNP improves the diagnostic evaluation of heart failure in older people when added to assessment of symptoms and signs [17]. However there are a few limitations to the use of BNP in older patients such as increase in levels related to advancing age, renal impairment and chronic obstructive pulmonary disease [18, 19]. In people aged >70 years, change of N-terminal-pro-Brain-Natriuretic Peptide (NT-proBNP) over time, correlates independently with all-cause and cardiovascular mortality [20].

CARDIORENAL SYNDROME

Heart failure and renal insufficiency frequently coexist and the term cardiorenal syndrome (CRS) is often used to describe this scenario. This syndrome is relevant to older people because increasing age is a risk factor [21]. In 2008, Ronco and colleagues presented a classification of CRS with five subgroups that reflect its pathophysiology and its bidirectional interaction between heart and kidney (Table 1) [22].

Table 1. Cardiorenal syndrome classification.

Type 1 – acute cardiorenal syndrome Rapid deterioration in cardiac function resulting in acute kidney injury. **Type 2** – chronic cardiorenal syndrome Chronic cardiac dysfunction leading to progressive chronic kidney disease. **Type 3** – acute renocardiac syndrome Primary and sudden deterioration in kidney function resulting in acute cardiac dysfunction **Type 4** – chronic renocardiac syndrome. Primary chronic kidney disease leading to decrease cardiac function, ventricular hypertrophy, diastolic dysfunction and/or adverse cardiovascular events. **Type 5** – secondary cardiorenal syndrome Combined cardiac and renal dysfunction arising from acute or chronic systemic disorders.

Adapted from Ronco C, *et al.* [22].

Current management strategies for CRS in older people are mainly focused on the correction of haemodynamic aberrations. Fluid balance is especially critical in the elderly: overfilling may lead to pulmonary oedema and underfilling may worsen kidney function. There are trials on BNP derivative [23], endothelin receptor antagonist [24] and vasopressin antagonist [25] in CRS but their effects have not been conclusive and older people are underrepresented. The use of ultrafiltration and peritoneal dialysis in patients with acute decompensated heart failure have produced variable results [26 - 28] but these approaches have not been evaluated in older people.

HEART FAILURE AND GERIATRIC SYNDROMES

Cognitive impairment is relatively common in older people with heart failure. Studies have reported a prevalence of at least 25% [29]. One study found that the prevalence of cognitive impairment is greater in heart failure patients with recent hospitalisation [30]. Another study reported that heart failure appeared to confer a high risk of cognitive impairment compared with other cardiovascular disorder

[31]. Cognitive impairment is independently associated with mortality in patients with heart failure [32]. Cognitive impairment may affect outcomes by impeding heart failure self-care such as symptom monitoring, medication adherence, dietary compliance and self-weighing [33].

Frailty which is defined as an increased physiological vulnerability to stressors [34] has a significant impact on older people. In a small study of 60 older patients with heart failure and ejection fraction <40%, frailty was present in 25% [35]. In women aged 65-79 years enrolled in the Women's Health Initiative Observational Study, participants with frailty were almost six times more likely to have heart failure compared with those without [36]. Several small studies of older people with heart failure have shown that frailty is independently associated with increased hospitalisation and mortality [37, 38].

Heart failure has been associated with increased risk of falls-related fractures in at least two studies [39, 40]. After hospitalisation for fractures, older people with heart failure have worse outcomes than those without heart failure [40, 41]. While there has been concern that beta-blockers may be associated with increased risk of falls, two meta-analyses have failed to show any association between this class of drug and falls [42, 43].

Urinary incontinence is a common problem in older adults with heart failure. One study of 269 patients (age ≥65 years) with heart failure found that 17.5% had urinary incontinence and the prevalence increased to 42.9% in those aged ≥85 years [44]. The most apparent link between heart failure and urinary incontinence is related to diuretic therapy, and it is likely to adversely affect adherence to these medications. One small study of incontinent older people found that 20 out of 21 who were prescribed diuretics did not take these drugs in an attempt to control their incontinence [45].

NON-PHARMACOLOGICAL MANAGEMENT

Regular physical activity is strongly encouraged in people with heart failure in order to reduce physical deconditioning and improve functional capacity. In patients with heart failure and LVEF ≤35%, The Heart Failure: A Controlled Trial Investigating Outcomes of Exercise Training (HF-ACTION) showed that aerobic exercise, in addition to standard care, improved self-reported health status including quality of life [46]. A retrospective analysis of the study (adjusted for prognostic factors) revealed that participants who exercised achieved modestly significant improvement in all-cause mortality or hospitalisation and cardiovascular-related mortality or hospitalisation for heart failure [47]. However there is still a lack of evidence to demonstrate the benefit of physical activity in older patients and those with HFPEF.

Salt and fluid restriction must be emphasized in all patients with heart failure, especially in those who are volume overloaded. For patients with mild symptoms (clinically stable, New York Heart Association, NYHA Class II and no peripheral oedema), it is suggested that limiting sodium intake to 3 g/day is sufficient to control extracellular fluid volume [48]. For patients with moderate to severe symptoms (NYHA Class III/IV) requiring a diuretic, a restricted intake of 2 g/day should be applied [48].

PHARMACOTHERAPY FOR HEART FAILURE WITH REDUCED EJECTION FRACTION

A large number of studies have shown that angiotensin converting-enzyme (ACE) inhibitors, angiotensin receptor blockers (ARB), beta-blockers and aldosterone antagonists reduced the mortality of HFREF patients. However, very few studies have focused on these therapies in older people with HFREF.

Available evidence indicates that the efficacy of ACE inhibitors and ARB in HFREF are similar in the younger and older people. A review of studies on ACE inhibitor use have found that the reduced mortality and hospitalization rates were consistent across all age subgroups and more evident in patients with LVEF <35% [49]. Another study has found that an ARB, candesartan, reduced hospitalization and cardiovascular mortality in patients with heart failure independent of age [50]. ARB seems to be better tolerated by older people than ACE inhibitors. The Evaluation of Losartan in The Elderly-II (ELITE II) study which compared losartan and captopril in patients aged >65 years with LVEF <40% and found the two drugs to be similarly effective but ARB was better tolerated [51].

Antagonism of the sympathetic nervous system overactivity is another important aspect in the treatment of HFREF. Meta-analyses of studies on beta-blocker use in HFREF have shown mortality and morbidity rates were reduced by 30% [52]. So far, the Study of Effects of Nebivolol Intervention on Outcomes and Rehospitalization in Seniors with Heart Failure (SENIORS) is the largest randomized trial investigating the efficacy of beta-blocker therapy in older people (enrolled people aged >70 years) [53]. This study showed that nebivolol reduced the composite endpoint of all-cause mortality and cardiovascular-related hospital admissions compared to placebo, but not cardiovascular mortality. These beneficial outcomes were observed after six months of treatment and the reduction of risk continued to increase with longer duration of treatment. Nonetheless, the benefits seem to be less in subjects aged >75 years. In addition, older patients on beta-blocker therapy had a higher risk of adverse effects compared to the younger age group [53].

Aldosterone antagonists, spironolactone and eplerenone, have also been shown to be beneficial in heart failure treatment. The Eplerenone in Mild Patients Hospitalization and Survival Study in Heart Failure (EMPHASIS-HF) showed that this drug reduced the risk of cardiovascular-related mortality and hospitalization for heart failure [54]. Furthermore, these results were not statistically different between older patients (≥75 years; 24% of study cohort) and those aged <75 years. However, in older adults with renal impairment, the risk of hyperkalaemia is increased with the use of aldosterone antagonists [55]. Therefore serum potassium and creatinine should be monitored closely in older patients started on an aldosterone antagonist. It should also be taken into consideration that spironolactone-related gynaecomastia is more common in older males [56].

Ivabradine is a direct sinus node inhibitor that inhibits the I_f channel in the sinus node. In patients with symptomatic systolic heart failure (LVEF <35%), sinus rhythm (heart rate ≥70 beats/min) and recent hospitalization with heart failure, ivabradine has been shown to reduce composite endpoint of cardiovascular mortality and hospitalization for heart failure (Hazard ratio: 0.82; 95% Confidence interval: 0.75-0.90; P <0.001) [57]. However no significant reduction in cardiovascular death alone and all-cause mortality was observed. Another important aspect of this study to note is that only 10% of the cohort was aged >70 years.

Digoxin can be used in low doses for patients who are symptomatic despite appropriate therapy with an ACE inhibitor or an ARB and a beta-blocker [58]. A daily dose of 125 microgram is often sufficient for most patients but monitoring of serum digoxin levels may be required for those with renal impairment.

Most older patients with heart failure need loop diuretics to achieve and maintain euvolemia [59]. Diuretics are known to activate neurohormones that are potentially harmful [60]. Once euvolemia has been achieved, diuretics should be used at the lowest possible dose to maintain this euvolemic state. In older people taking long-term diuretics, a close monitoring of their hydration status and electrolyte levels is required. In addition, when it is difficult to reach a balance between volume status and renal insufficiency, it could be reasonable to accept some degree of volume overload with slight worsening of renal function [61].

In patients with heart failure, there are a number of medications that should be avoided such as non-steroidal anti-inflammatory drugs (NSAIDs), cyclo-oxygenase-2 (COX-2) inhibitors, thiazolidinediones, tyrosine kinase inhibitors and moxonidine [62 - 64]. Some of these medications such as NSAIDs and COX-2 inhibitors are commonly prescribed to older people or obtained over-the-counter for treatment of pain.

DEVICES IN HEART FAILURE WITH REDUCED EJECTION FRACTION

Current guidelines recommend an implantable cardioverter-defibrillator (ICD) to prevent sudden death in patients with HFREF [59]. However a meta-analysis of three large trials has not shown a significant survival benefit with the prophylactic implantation of ICD in older people [65]. Furthermore one meta-analysis of ICD in women with advanced heart failure for primary prevention of sudden cardiac death found that morbidity and mortality rates were higher in patients older than 80 years [66]. As result the need for an ICD in older people with heart failure is still debated. An important consideration for ICD in older people relates to its influence on quality of life, especially those with severe or terminal non-cardiac diseases. In some patients at the terminal stage of diseases and death is estimated to be near, the deactivation of ICD can be an appropriate measure after careful discussion of all legal and ethical issues on the matter [67, 68].

For patients already on optimal medical therapy, cardiac resynchronization therapy (CRT) can reverse ventricular remodelling, improve functional capacity, and clinical outcome in advanced chronic heart failure with reduced ejection fraction, and evidence of ventricular conduction delay [69]. An observational study found that patients aged >80 years, 70-79 years and <70 years, had similar improvement in left ventricular remodelling and functional capacity after undergoing CRT [70]. However patients aged >80 years still have a higher annual mortality in this study. CRT could be considered an effective strategy to improve the quality of life for older patients with heart failure. Like ICD, its use in the older population needs to be weighed against the presence of coexisting comorbidities and estimated life expectancy.

In patients with heart failure and symptomatic recurrent atrial fibrillation despite conventional therapy, catheter ablation may be indicated for symptom improvement (European Heart Rhythm Association score II-IV) [71]. Nonrandomized studies involving drug-refractory symptomatic AF patients showed that complication rates was no different between younger patients and those aged >65 years [72]. In this same study, even those aged ≥80 years had similar periprocedural complications as the younger cohorts [72]. Nonetheless, randomised controlled trials are still needed to verify the long-term efficacy of ablation therapy in older patients. In selected patients, ablation of the atrioventricular node and ventricular pacing should be considered when pharmacological rate and rhythm control has failed with a combination of medications [73].

PHARMACOTHERAPY FOR HEART FAILURE WITH PRESERVED EJECTION FRACTION

In contrast to HFREF, no controlled randomised trial has shown any improvement in survival of patients with HFPEF. Trials that tested the efficacy of a therapeutic approach based on inhibition of the neurohormonal system has failed to show any benefit in reducing mortality of HFPEF [74 - 76]. Preliminary results have suggested that an aldosterone antagonist could be useful in improving diastolic dysfunction but this approach is still under further investigation [77]. The Treatment of Preserved Cardiac Function Heart Failure With an Aldosterone Antagonist (TOP-CAT) study is currently ongoing and is intended to evaluate the use of spironolactone in HFPEF [78]. The absence of demonstrated benefit from existing therapeutic approaches strengthens the need for new trials to define the best way to manage HFPEF.

GAPS IN EVIDENCE

Evidence is still lacking about the most effective diagnostic and therapeutic approaches to use in older people with heart failure. The dearth of evidence is even more apparent in HFPEF which affects a large proportion of older people. There is limited data on the cost-effectiveness of device therapies in the elderly population and which older individuals should be selected to receive such devices.

CONCLUSION

Heart failure has a high prevalence among the older population. The diagnostic and therapeutic approach to heart failure especially HFPEF is still challenging in this group of patients. In older people with heart failure, it is important also to assess and manage associated geriatric syndromes. Further interventional studies that focus on older people with heart failure are required to better guide management.

CONFLICT OF INTEREST

The author confirms that author has no conflict of interest to declare for this publication.

ACKNOWLEDGEMENTS

Declared none.

KEY POINTS

- With population ageing, heart failure is a major and growing health problem among older people.
- Diagnosis of heart failure in the older people is challenging because of

comorbidities mimicking or masking clinical features of heart failure.

- Geriatric syndromes such as cognitive impairment, frailty, falls and urinary incontinence are common among older people with heart failure and can influence patients' prognosis.

REFERENCES

[1] Schocken DD, Arrieta MI, Leaverton PE, Ross EA. Prevalence and mortality rate of congestive heart failure in the United States. J Am Coll Cardiol 1992; 20(2): 301-6. [http://dx.doi.org/10.1016/0735-1097(92)90094-4] [PMID: 1634664]

[2] Forman DE, Ahmed A, Fleg JL. Heart failure in very old adults. Curr Heart Fail Rep 2013; 10(4): 387-400. [http://dx.doi.org/10.1007/s11897-013-0163-7] [PMID: 24091808]

[3] Jessup M, Abraham WT, Casey DE, *et al.* 2009 focused update: ACCF/AHA guidelines for the diagnosis and management of heart failure in adults: a report of the American college of cardiology foundation/American heart association task force on practice guidelines: developed in collaboration with the international society for heart and lung transplantation. Circulation 2009; 119(14): 1977-2016. [http://dx.doi.org/10.1161/CIRCULATIONAHA.109.192064] [PMID: 19324967]

[4] Ahmed A, Allman RM, Aronow WS, DeLong JF. Diagnosis of heart failure in older adults: predictive value of dyspnea at rest. Arch Gerontol Geriatr 2004; 38(3): 297-307. [http://dx.doi.org/10.1016/j.archger.2003.12.001] [PMID: 15066316]

[5] Wang CS, FitzGerald JM, Schulzer M, Mak E, Ayas NT. Does this dyspneic patient in the emergency department have congestive heart failure? JAMA 2005; 294(15): 1944-56. [http://dx.doi.org/10.1001/jama.294.15.1944] [PMID: 16234501]

[6] Butman SM, Ewy GA, Standen JR, Kern KB, Hahn E. Bedside cardiovascular examination in patients with severe chronic heart failure: importance of rest or inducible jugular venous distension. J Am Coll Cardiol 1993; 22(4): 968-74. [http://dx.doi.org/10.1016/0735-1097(93)90405-P] [PMID: 8409071]

[7] Drazner MH, Rame JE, Stevenson LW, Dries DL. Prognostic importance of elevated jugular venous pressure and a third heart sound in patients with heart failure. N Engl J Med 2001; 345(8): 574-81. [http://dx.doi.org/10.1056/NEJMoa010641] [PMID: 11529211]

[8] Kannel WB. Vital epidemiologic clues in heart failure. J Clin Epidemiol 2000; 53(3): 229-35. [http://dx.doi.org/10.1016/S0895-4356(99)00135-3] [PMID: 10760631]

[9] Gottdiener JS, Arnold AM, Aurigemma GP, *et al.* Predictors of congestive heart failure in the elderly: the Cardiovascular Health Study. J Am Coll Cardiol 2000; 35(6): 1628-37. [http://dx.doi.org/10.1016/S0735-1097(00)00582-9] [PMID: 10807470]

[10] Gottdiener JS, McClelland RL, Marshall R, *et al.* Outcome of congestive heart failure in elderly persons: influence of left ventricular systolic function. The Cardiovascular Health Study. Ann Intern Med 2002; 137(8): 631-9. [http://dx.doi.org/10.7326/0003-4819-137-8-200210150-00006] [PMID: 12379062]

[11] McMurray JJ. Clinical practice. Systolic heart failure. N Engl J Med 2010; 362(3): 228-38. [http://dx.doi.org/10.1056/NEJMcp0909392] [PMID: 20089973]

[12] Hogg K, Swedberg K, McMurray J. Heart failure with preserved left ventricular systolic function; epidemiology, clinical characteristics, and prognosis. J Am Coll Cardiol 2004; 43(3): 317-27. [http://dx.doi.org/10.1016/j.jacc.2003.07.046] [PMID: 15013109]

[13] Senni M, Redfield MM. Heart failure with preserved systolic function. A different natural history? J Am Coll Cardiol 2001; 38(5): 1277-82. [http://dx.doi.org/10.1016/S0735-1097(01)01567-4] [PMID: 11691495]

[14] Zile MR, Gaasch WH, Carroll JD, *et al.* Heart failure with a normal ejection fraction: is measurement of diastolic function necessary to make the diagnosis of diastolic heart failure? Circulation 2001; 104(7): 779-82. [http://dx.doi.org/10.1161/hc3201.094226] [PMID: 11502702]

[15] Ahmed A. Association of diastolic dysfunction and outcomes in ambulatory older adults with chronic heart failure. J Gerontol A Biol Sci Med Sci 2005; 60(10): 1339-44. [http://dx.doi.org/10.1093/gerona/60.10.1339] [PMID: 16282571]

[16] Maisel A, Mueller C, Adams K Jr, *et al.* State of the art: using natriuretic peptide levels in clinical practice. Eur J Heart Fail 2008; 10(9): 824-39. [http://dx.doi.org/10.1016/j.ejheart.2008.07.014] [PMID: 18760965]

[17] Jensen J, Ma LP, Bjurman C, Hammarsten O, Fu ML. Prognostic values of NTpro BNP/BNP ratio in comparison with NTpro BNP or BNP alone in elderly patients with chronic heart failure in a 2-year follow up. Int J Cardiol 2012; 155(1): 1-5. [http://dx.doi.org/10.1016/j.ijcard.2011.01.083] [PMID: 21334085]

[18] Wang TJ, Larson MG, Levy D, *et al.* Impact of age and sex on plasma natriuretic peptide levels in healthy adults. Am J Cardiol 2002; 90(3): 254-8. [http://dx.doi.org/10.1016/S0002-9149(02)02464-5] [PMID: 12127613]

[19] Vaes B, Gruson D, Van Pottelbergh G, *et al.* The impact of confounders on the test performance of natriuretic peptides for cardiac dysfunction in subjects aged 80 and older. Peptides 2012; 38(1): 118-26. [http://dx.doi.org/10.1016/j.peptides.2012.08.020] [PMID: 22986019]

[20] Eggers KM, Venge P, Lind L. Prognostic usefulness of the change in N-terminal pro B-type natriuretic peptide levels to predict mortality in a single community cohort aged ≥ 70 years. Am J Cardiol 2013; 111(1): 131-6. [http://dx.doi.org/10.1016/j.amjcard.2012.08.058] [PMID: 23040598]

[21] Shlipak MG, Massie BM. The clinical challenge of cardiorenal syndrome. Circulation 2004; 110(12): 1514-7. [http://dx.doi.org/10.1161/01.CIR.0000143547.55093.17] [PMID: 15381655]

[22] Ronco C, Haapio M, House AA, Anavekar N, Bellomo R. Cardiorenal syndrome. J Am Coll Cardiol 2008; 52(19): 1527-39. [http://dx.doi.org/10.1016/j.jacc.2008.07.051] [PMID: 19007588]

[23] Elkayam U, Janmohamed M, Hatamizadeh P, Heywood JT, Wei LJ, Mills RM. Impact of acute serum

creatinine elevation in patients treated with nesiritide. Clin Cardiol 2009; 32(4): 215-9. [http://dx.doi.org/10.1002/clc.20344] [PMID: 19353723]

[24] McMurray JJ, Teerlink JR, Cotter G, *et al.* Effects of tezosentan on symptoms and clinical outcomes in patients with acute heart failure: the VERITAS randomized controlled trials. JAMA 2007; 298(17): 2009-19.
[http://dx.doi.org/10.1001/jama.298.17.2009] [PMID: 17986694]

[25] Konstam MA, Gheorghiade M, Burnett JC Jr, *et al.* Effects of oral tolvaptan in patients hospitalized for worsening heart failure: the EVEREST Outcome Trial. JAMA 2007; 297(12): 1319-31.
[http://dx.doi.org/10.1001/jama.297.12.1319] [PMID: 17384437]

[26] Bertoli SV, Ciurlino D, Maccario M, *et al.* Home peritoneal ultrafiltration in patients with severe congestive heart failure without end-stage renal disease. Adv Perit Dial 2005; 21: 123-7.
[PMID: 16686301]

[27] Costanzo MR, Guglin ME, Saltzberg MT, *et al.* Ultrafiltration *versus* intravenous diuretics for patients hospitalized for acute decompensated heart failure. J Am Coll Cardiol 2007; 49(6): 675-83.
[http://dx.doi.org/10.1016/j.jacc.2006.07.073] [PMID: 17291932]

[28] Bart BA, Goldsmith SR, Lee KL, *et al.* Ultrafiltration in decompensated heart failure with cardiorenal syndrome. N Engl J Med 2012; 367(24): 2296-304.
[http://dx.doi.org/10.1056/NEJMoa1210357] [PMID: 23131078]

[29] Vogels RL, Scheltens P, Schroeder-Tanka JM, Weinstein HC. Cognitive impairment in heart failure: a systematic review of the literature. Eur J Heart Fail 2007; 9(5): 440-9.
[http://dx.doi.org/10.1016/j.ejheart.2006.11.001] [PMID: 17174152]

[30] Harkness K, Demers C, Heckman GA, McKelvie RS. Screening for cognitive deficits using the Montreal cognitive assessment tool in outpatients ≥65 years of age with heart failure. Am J Cardiol 2011; 107(8): 1203-7.
[http://dx.doi.org/10.1016/j.amjcard.2010.12.021] [PMID: 21310371]

[31] Vogels RL, Oosterman JM, van Harten B, *et al.* Profile of cognitive impairment in chronic heart failure. J Am Geriatr Soc 2007; 55(11): 1764-70.
[http://dx.doi.org/10.1111/j.1532-5415.2007.01395.x] [PMID: 17727641]

[32] Chaudhry SI, Wang Y, Gill TM, Krumholz HM. Geriatric conditions and subsequent mortality in older patients with heart failure. J Am Coll Cardiol 2010; 55(4): 309-16.
[http://dx.doi.org/10.1016/j.jacc.2009.07.066] [PMID: 20117435]

[33] Dickson VV, Tkacs N, Riegel B. Cognitive influences on self-care decision making in persons with heart failure. Am Heart J 2007; 154(3): 424-31.
[http://dx.doi.org/10.1016/j.ahj.2007.04.058] [PMID: 17719284]

[34] Fried LP, Tangen CM, Walston J, *et al.* Frailty in older adults: evidence for a phenotype. J Gerontol A Biol Sci Med Sci 2001; 56(3): M146-56.
[http://dx.doi.org/10.1093/gerona/56.3.M146] [PMID: 11253156]

[35] Boxer RS, Wang Z, Walsh SJ, Hager D, Kenny AM. The utility of the 6-minute walk test as a measure of frailty in older adults with heart failure. Am J Geriatr Cardiol 2008; 17(1): 7-12.
[http://dx.doi.org/10.1111/j.1076-7460.2007.06457.x] [PMID: 18174754]

[36] Woods NF, LaCroix AZ, Gray SL, *et al.* Frailty: emergence and consequences in women aged 65 and older in the Women's Health Initiative Observational Study. J Am Geriatr Soc 2005; 53(8): 1321-30. [http://dx.doi.org/10.1111/j.1532-5415.2005.53405.x] [PMID: 16078957]

[37] Cacciatore F, Abete P, Mazzella F, *et al.* Frailty predicts long-term mortality in elderly subjects with chronic heart failure. Eur J Clin Invest 2005; 35(12): 723-30. [http://dx.doi.org/10.1111/j.1365-2362.2005.01572.x] [PMID: 16313247]

[38] Boxer R, Kleppinger A, Ahmad A, Annis K, Hager D, Kenny A. The 6-minute walk is associated with frailty and predicts mortality in older adults with heart failure. Congest Heart Fail 2010; 16(5): 208-13. [http://dx.doi.org/10.1111/j.1751-7133.2010.00151.x] [PMID: 20887617]

[39] van Diepen S, Majumdar SR, Bakal JA, McAlister FA, Ezekowitz JA. Heart failure is a risk factor for orthopedic fracture: a population-based analysis of 16,294 patients. Circulation 2008; 118(19): 1946-52. [http://dx.doi.org/10.1161/CIRCULATIONAHA.108.784009] [PMID: 18936331]

[40] Cullen MW, Gullerud RE, Larson DR, Melton LJ III, Huddleston JM. Impact of heart failure on hip fracture outcomes: a population-based study. J Hosp Med 2011; 6(9): 507-12. [http://dx.doi.org/10.1002/jhm.918] [PMID: 22042721]

[41] Kannegaard PN, van der Mark S, Eiken P, Abrahamsen B. Excess mortality in men compared with women following a hip fracture. National analysis of comedications, comorbidity and survival. Age Ageing 2010; 39(2): 203-9. [http://dx.doi.org/10.1093/ageing/afp221] [PMID: 20075035]

[42] Leipzig RM, Cumming RG, Tinetti ME. Drugs and falls in older people: a systematic review and meta-analysis: II. Cardiac and analgesic drugs. J Am Geriatr Soc 1999; 47(1): 40-50. [http://dx.doi.org/10.1111/j.1532-5415.1999.tb01899.x] [PMID: 9920228]

[43] Woolcott JC, Richardson KJ, Wiens MO, *et al.* Meta-analysis of the impact of 9 medication classes on falls in elderly persons. Arch Intern Med 2009; 169(21): 1952-60. [http://dx.doi.org/10.1001/archinternmed.2009.357] [PMID: 19933955]

[44] van der Wel MC, Jansen RW, Bakx JC, Bor HH, Olderikkert MG, van Weel C. Non-cardiovascular co-morbidity in elderly patients with heart failure outnumbers cardiovascular co-morbidity. Eur J Heart Fail 2007; 9(6-7): 709-15. [http://dx.doi.org/10.1016/j.ejheart.2007.02.004] [PMID: 17395533]

[45] McKeever MP. An investigation of recognized incontinence within a health authority. J Adv Nurs 1990; 15(10): 1197-207. [http://dx.doi.org/10.1111/j.1365-2648.1990.tb01713.x] [PMID: 2258528]

[46] Flynn KE, Piña IL, Whellan DJ, *et al.* Effects of exercise training on health status in patients with chronic heart failure: HF-ACTION randomized controlled trial. JAMA 2009; 301(14): 1451-9. [http://dx.doi.org/10.1001/jama.2009.457] [PMID: 19351942]

[47] O'Connor CM, Whellan DJ, Lee KL, *et al.* Efficacy and safety of exercise training in patients with chronic heart failure: HF-ACTION randomized controlled trial. JAMA 2009; 301(14): 1439-50. [http://dx.doi.org/10.1001/jama.2009.454] [PMID: 19351941]

[48] Dracup K, Baker DW, Dunbar SB, *et al.* Management of heart failure. II. Counseling, education, and

lifestyle modifications. JAMA 1994; 272(18): 1442-6.
[http://dx.doi.org/10.1001/jama.1994.03520180066037] [PMID: 7933427]

[49] Garg R, Yusuf S. Overview of randomized trials of angiotensin-converting enzyme inhibitors on mortality and morbidity in patients with heart failure. JAMA 1995; 273(18): 1450-6.
[http://dx.doi.org/10.1001/jama.1995.03520420066040] [PMID: 7654275]

[50] Cohen-Solal A, McMurray JJ, Swedberg K, *et al.* Benefits and safety of candesartan treatment in heart failure are independent of age: insights from the Candesartan in Heart failure--Assessment of Reduction in Mortality and morbidity programme. Eur Heart J 2008; 29(24): 3022-8.
[http://dx.doi.org/10.1093/eurheartj/ehn476] [PMID: 18987098]

[51] Pitt B, Poole-Wilson PA, Segal R, *et al.* Effect of losartan compared with captopril on mortality in patients with symptomatic heart failure: randomised trial--the Losartan Heart Failure Survival Study ELITE II. Lancet 2000; 355(9215): 1582-7.
[http://dx.doi.org/10.1016/S0140-6736(00)02213-3] [PMID: 10821361]

[52] Brophy JM, Joseph L, Rouleau JL. Beta-blockers in congestive heart failure. A Bayesian meta-analysis. Ann Intern Med 2001; 134(7): 550-60.
[http://dx.doi.org/10.7326/0003-4819-134-7-200104030-00008] [PMID: 11281737]

[53] Flather MD, Shibata MC, Coats AJ, *et al.* Randomized trial to determine the effect of nebivolol on mortality and cardiovascular hospital admission in elderly patients with heart failure (SENIORS). Eur Heart J 2005; 26(3): 215-25.
[http://dx.doi.org/10.1093/eurheartj/ehi115] [PMID: 15642700]

[54] Zannad F, McMurray JJ, Krum H, *et al.* Eplerenone in patients with systolic heart failure and mild symptoms. N Engl J Med 2011; 364(1): 11-21.
[http://dx.doi.org/10.1056/NEJMoa1009492] [PMID: 21073363]

[55] Juurlink DN, Mamdani MM, Lee DS, *et al.* Rates of hyperkalemia after publication of the Randomized Aldactone Evaluation Study. N Engl J Med 2004; 351(6): 543-51.
[http://dx.doi.org/10.1056/NEJMoa040135] [PMID: 15295047]

[56] Braunstein GD. Clinical practice. Gynecomastia. N Engl J Med 2007; 357(12): 1229-37.
[http://dx.doi.org/10.1056/NEJMcp070677] [PMID: 17881754]

[57] Swedberg K, Komajda M, Böhm M, *et al.* Ivabradine and outcomes in chronic heart failure (SHIFT): a randomised placebo-controlled study. Lancet 2010; 376(9744): 875-85.
[http://dx.doi.org/10.1016/S0140-6736(10)61198-1] [PMID: 20801500]

[58] Ahmed A, Rich MW, Love TE, *et al.* Digoxin and reduction in mortality and hospitalization in heart failure: a comprehensive post hoc analysis of the DIG trial. Eur Heart J 2006; 27(2): 178-86.
[http://dx.doi.org/10.1093/eurheartj/ehi687] [PMID: 16339157]

[59] McMurray JJ, Adamopoulos S, Anker SD, *et al.* ESC guidelines for the diagnosis and treatment of acute and chronic heart failure 2012: The task force for the diagnosis and treatment of acute and chronic heart failure 2012 of the European society of cardiology. developed in collaboration with the heart failure association (HFA) of the ESC. Eur J Heart Fail 2012; 14(8): 803-69.
[http://dx.doi.org/10.1093/eurjhf/hfs105] [PMID: 22828712]

[60] Ahmed A, Young JB, Love TE, Levesque R, Pitt B. A propensity-matched study of the effects of

chronic diuretic therapy on mortality and hospitalization in older adults with heart failure. Int J Cardiol 2008; 125(2): 246-53.
[http://dx.doi.org/10.1016/j.ijcard.2007.05.032] [PMID: 17706809]

[61] Rich MW. Pharmacotherapy of heart failure in the elderly: adverse events. Heart Fail Rev 2012; 17(4-5): 589-95.
[http://dx.doi.org/10.1007/s10741-011-9263-1] [PMID: 21688185]

[62] Krum H, Jelinek MV, Stewart S, Sindone A, Atherton JJ. 2011 update to National Heart Foundation of Australia and Cardiac Society of Australia and New Zealand Guidelines for the prevention, detection and management of chronic heart failure in Australia, 2006. Med J Aust 2011; 194(8): 405-9.
[PMID: 21495941]

[63] Krum H, Jelinek MV, Stewart S, Sindone A, Atherton JJ, Hawkes AL. Guidelines for the prevention, detection and management of people with chronic heart failure in Australia 2006. Med J Aust 2006; 185(10): 549-57.
[PMID: 17115967]

[64] Page K, Marwick TH, Lee R, *et al.* A systematic approach to chronic heart failure care: a consensus statement. Med J Aust 2014; 201(3): 146-50.
[http://dx.doi.org/10.5694/mja14.00032] [PMID: 25128948]

[65] Santangeli P, Di Biase L, Dello Russo A, *et al.* Meta-analysis: age and effectiveness of prophylactic implantable cardioverter-defibrillators. Ann Intern Med 2010; 153(9): 592-9.
[http://dx.doi.org/10.7326/0003-4819-153-9-201011020-00009] [PMID: 21041579]

[66] Ghanbari H, Dalloul G, Hasan R, *et al.* Effectiveness of implantable cardioverter-defibrillators for the primary prevention of sudden cardiac death in women with advanced heart failure: a meta-analysis of randomized controlled trials. Arch Intern Med 2009; 169(16): 1500-6.
[http://dx.doi.org/10.1001/archinternmed.2009.255] [PMID: 19752408]

[67] Revenco D, Morgan JP, Tsao L. The dilemma of implantable cardioverter-defibrillator therapy in the geriatric population. J Geriatr Cardiol 2011; 8(3): 195-200.
[http://dx.doi.org/10.3724/SP.J.1263.2011.00195] [PMID: 22783305]

[68] Padeletti L, Arnar DO, Boncinelli L, *et al.* EHRA Expert Consensus Statement on the management of cardiovascular implantable electronic devices in patients nearing end of life or requesting withdrawal of therapy. Europace 2010; 12(10): 1480-9.
[http://dx.doi.org/10.1093/europace/euq275] [PMID: 20675674]

[69] McAlister FA, Ezekowitz J, Hooton N, *et al.* Cardiac resynchronization therapy for patients with left ventricular systolic dysfunction: a systematic review. JAMA 2007; 297(22): 2502-14.
[http://dx.doi.org/10.1001/jama.297.22.2502] [PMID: 17565085]

[70] Verbrugge FH, Dupont M, De Vusser P, *et al.* Response to cardiac resynchronization therapy in elderly patients (≥70 years) and octogenarians. Eur J Heart Fail 2013; 15(2): 203-10.
[http://dx.doi.org/10.1093/eurjhf/hfs151] [PMID: 23002114]

[71] Camm AJ, Lip GY, De Caterina R, *et al.* 2012 focused update of the ESC Guidelines for the management of atrial fibrillation: an update of the 2010 ESC Guidelines for the management of atrial fibrillation. Developed with the special contribution of the European Heart Rhythm Association. Eur Heart J 2012; 33(21): 2719-47.

[http://dx.doi.org/10.1093/eurheartj/ehs253] [PMID: 22922413]

[72] Haegeli LM, Duru F. Management of patients with atrial fibrillation: specific considerations for the old age Cardiol Res Pract 2011; 2011: 854205.
[http://dx.doi.org/10.4061/2011/854205]

[73] Haegeli LM, Duru F. Atrial fibrillation in the aging heart: pharmacological therapy and catheter ablation in the elderly. Future Cardiol 2011; 7(3): 415-23.
[http://dx.doi.org/10.2217/fca.11.22] [PMID: 21627480]

[74] Cleland JG, Tendera M, Adamus J, Freemantle N, Polonski L, Taylor J. The perindopril in elderly people with chronic heart failure (PEP-CHF) study. Eur Heart J 2006; 27(19): 2338-45.
[http://dx.doi.org/10.1093/eurheartj/ehl250] [PMID: 16963472]

[75] Yusuf S, Pfeffer MA, Swedberg K, *et al.* Effects of candesartan in patients with chronic heart failure and preserved left-ventricular ejection fraction: the CHARM-Preserved Trial. Lancet 2003; 362(9386): 777-81.
[http://dx.doi.org/10.1016/S0140-6736(03)14285-7] [PMID: 13678871]

[76] Massie BM, Carson PE, McMurray JJ, *et al.* Irbesartan in patients with heart failure and preserved ejection fraction. N Engl J Med 2008; 359(23): 2456-67.
[http://dx.doi.org/10.1056/NEJMoa0805450] [PMID: 19001508]

[77] Mottram PM, Haluska B, Leano R, Cowley D, Stowasser M, Marwick TH. Effect of aldosterone antagonism on myocardial dysfunction in hypertensive patients with diastolic heart failure. Circulation 2004; 110(5): 558-65.
[http://dx.doi.org/10.1161/01.CIR.0000138680.89536.A9] [PMID: 15277317]

[78] Desai AS, Lewis EF, Li R, Solomon SD, Assmann SF, Boineau R, *et al.* Rationale and design of the treatment of preserved cardiac function heart failure with an aldosterone antagonist trial: a randomized, controlled study of spironolactone in patients with symptomatic heart failure and preserved ejection fraction. Am Heart J 2011; 162(6): 966-72.
[http://dx.doi.org/10.1016/j.ahj.2011.09.007]

Recent Advances in Geriatric Medicine, 2016, *Vol. 1*, 34-49

CHAPTER 3

Updates on Treating Hypertension in Older People

Danielle Wu[1], Kareeann Sok Fun Khow[2,*]

[1] *Department of Nephrology, Mackay Base Hospital, Mackay, Queensland, Australia*

[2] *Aged and Extended Care Services, The Queen Elizabeth Hospital and Department of Medicine, University of Adelaide, Adelaide, South Australia, Australia*

Abstract: Our population is ageing, and as older people (≥65 years of age) are affected by hypertension, these individuals are at increased risk of organ damage or cardiovascular disease (CVD). They pose many management dilemmas because most hypertension trials had upper age limits with participant recruitment or did not present age-specific results. Because evidence-based guidelines have limited information on managing older patients with hypertension, recommendations are mostly based on expert opinion. Drug treatment for elderly hypertensive patients are generally recommended but with a greater degree of caution because of changes in drug distribution and elimination, as well as the need to consider quality of life factors. However, patients in most hypertension trials were aged <80 years. Pooling the limited number of octogenarians from several trials, this group of treated patients showed a reduction in both stroke and cardiovascular (CV) morbidity, but a trend toward higher all-cause mortality compared to controls.

Therefore, the overall benefits of lowering the blood pressure in octogenarians remain unclear despite epidemiological evidence that hypertension remains a major CV risk factor in this age group. Resistant hypertension (*i.e.*, blood pressure that remains above target when patient adheres to lifestyle measures and maximum tolerated doses of complementary antihypertensive agents which usually includes a diuretic) is more frequent with advancing age. Older patients with higher baseline systolic blood pressure characteristically have more severe or longer duration of hypertension, resulting in more difficult blood pressure control because it is often associated with autonomic dysfunction and organ damage.

* **Correspondence author Kareeann Sok Fun Khow:** Aged and Extended Care Services, The Queen Elizabeth Hospital, Woodville Road, Woodville South, South Australia 5011, Australia; Tel: +61 8 8222 6000; Fax: +61 8 8222 8178; E-mail: kareeann.khow@adelaide.edu.au.

Tuck Yean Yong (Ed)

Keywords: Angiotensin-converting enzyme inhibitors, Antihypertensives, Beta-blockers, Calcium channel antagonists, Cardiovascular diseases, Denervation of renal artery, Diuretic, Elderly, Hypertension.

INTRODUCTION

Hypertension is defined as a systolic blood pressure (SBP) of ≥140 mmHg or diastolic blood pressure (DBP) of ≥90 mmHg. Isolated hypertension is a SBP of ≥140 mmHg with a DBP of <90 mmHg [1]. Stage 1 hypertension is SBP of 140-159 mmHg with DBP of 90-99 mmHg while stage 2 is SBP of ≥160 mmHg or DBP of ≥100 mmHg [1]. Prehypertension is defined as SBP of 120-139 mmHg with DBP of 80-89 mmHg [1]. Resistant hypertension is defined as resistance to lower SBP and DBP values below 140 and 90 mm Hg, respectively, despite the use of three optimally dosed antihypertensive drugs from different classes with one of the medications being a diuretic [2].

The prevalence increases significantly with age, such that about two-thirds of those aged >60 years have hypertension [3]. Hypertension is a major risk factor for cardiovascular (CV) disease in older people. Hypertension is present in 69% of patients with a first myocardial infarct [4], 77% of those with a first stroke [4], 74% of those with heart failure [4] and 60% of those with peripheral vascular disease [5].

PATHOPHYSIOLOGY

Most cases of hypertension are caused by reduced elasticity and compliance of large arteries arising from ageing and from the atherosclerosis-associated accumulation of arterial calcium and collagen as well as arterial elastin degradation. Loss of arterial elasticity causes an elevation in the rate of return of reflected arterial pressure waves from the periphery, hence increasing the peak systolic pressure [6]. Rise in blood pressure (BP) itself can lead to further arterial stiffening and impairment in endothelium-dependent vasodilatation [7, 8].

EVALUATION

Assessment of an older person with hypertension should include evaluation for the presence of other CV risk factors, potentially contributing lifestyle factors, end-organ damage, and concomitant diseases affecting prognosis and treatment [9]. Physical examination must include evaluation of optic fundi, thyroid, heart, lungs, kidneys, peripheral pulses and the neurological systems. In rare situations, peripheral arteries can become so rigid that measuring BP with the standard arm cuff may lead to overestimating arterial pressure because of incomplete compression of the brachial artery [10]. Pseudohypertension should be considered when patients' blood pressure do not respond to therapy as expected or who have postural symptoms with treatment.

Laboratory tests and electrocardiography should be performed to evaluate CV risk and end-organ damage. Laboratory tests should include urinalysis, blood glucose, serum potassium, estimated glomerular filtration rate and lipid profile. Evidence of target organ damage will support a diagnosis of suboptimally-controlled BP and may affect decisions about appropriate treatment selection.

In patients with persistent office hypertension but no end-organ damage, ambulatory BP monitoring is recommended to determine if white-coat hypertension is contributory. Ambulatory BP monitoring is indicated when the diagnosis of hypertension or response to therapy is unclear from office visits, when syncope or hypotensive disorders are suspected, and symptoms of vertigo or dizziness require evaluation.

BLOOD PRESSURE GOALS IN OLDER PEOPLE

The American Academy of Neurology, the American Geriatrics Society, the American Society of Preventive Cardiology, the American Society of Hypertension, the American Society of Nephrology, the Association of Black Cardiologists and the European Society of Hypertension, the American College of Cardiology Foundation and American Heart Association (ACCF/AHA) 2011 expert consensus on hypertension in the elderly recommended that the SBP be reduced to <140 mmHg in older persons of less than 80 years and to 140-145 mmHg if tolerated in those aged 80 years or older [1]. These guidelines were based on data from the Systolic Hypertension in Elderly Program (SHEP) [11 - 13] and Hypertension in the Very Elderly (HYVET) [14] trials.

The European Society of Hypertension and European Society of Cardiology 2013 guidelines for management of hypertension recommended reducing the SBP to <140 mmHg in patients with low to moderate CV risk, diabetes mellitus, a prior stroke or transient ischaemic attack, coronary artery disease, and chronic kidney disease [15]. In older patients <80 years of age with a SBP of ≥160 mmHg, the SBP should be lowered to 140-150 mmHg if low to moderate CV risk is present with consideration of SBP <140 mmHg if concomitant vascular diseases are present [15]. In patients >80 years of age with SBP ≥160 mmHg, the SBP should be reduced to 140-150 mmHg provided they are in good physical and mental health [15].

The Eight Joint National Committee (JNC 8) guidelines for management of hypertension recommended reducing the SBP to <150 mmHg in patients aged ≥60 years if they do not have diabetes mellitus or chronic kidney disease and to <140 mmHg if these comorbidities are present [9].

BENEFITS OF BLOOD PRESSURE CONTROL IN OLDER PEOPLE

A meta-analysis of eight trials were undertaken, which included 15,693 patients aged ≥60 years with isolated hypertension who were followed for a median of 3-8 years [16]. The analysis found that antihypertensive therapy reduced all-cause mortality by 13% ($p = 0.02$), CV mortality by 18% ($p = 0.01$), CV events by 23% ($p < 0.0001$), stroke by 30% ($p < 0.001$) and acute coronary events by 23% ($p = 0.001$). The number needed to treat (NNT) to prevent one major CV event was 18 men compared to 38 women, and 19 persons aged ≥70 years of age compared to 39 persons <70 years [16].

Several antihypertensive trials [11, 14, 17 - 19] have demonstrated that drug therapy reduces CV events in older people younger than 89 years (Table **1**). The Systolic Hypertension in Elderly Program (SHEP) is a double-blind study which randomized 4736 patients (mean age 71.6 years; 14% aged ≥80 years) with isolated hypertension to antihypertensive therapy or placebo [11]. The primary outcome of stroke was reduced by 36% in the drug therapy group. The NNT to prevent one episode of stroke in 5 years was 33 persons [11]. In this study, major CV events were reduced by 32% in the drug therapy group which means that 18 persons needed to be treated to prevent one major CV event in 5 years [11].

Table 1. Summary of important clinical trials on hypertension in older people.

Study (Year)	Number	Inclusion Criteria	Blood Pressure Target	Antihypertensive Drugs	Main Outcomes
SHEP (1991)	4736	Age: ≥60 years (mean 71.6) BP 160-219/<90 mmHg	SBP <160 mmHg (if SBP ≥180 mmHg) or decrease by 20 mmHg (if SBP 160-179 mmHg)	Step 1: Chlorthalidone 12.5-25 mg daily Step 2: Atenolol 25-50 mg or reserpine 0.05-0.10 mg daily	Significant reduction in CV events (32%) and strokes (33%) but no reduction in all-cause mortality
STOP (1991)	1627	Age: 70-84 years (mean 75.6) BP 180-230/≥90 mmHg or DBP 105-20 mmHg	<160/<95 mmHg	Step 1: Atenolol 50 mg or HCTZ 25 mg + amiloride 2.5 mg or metoprolol 100 mg or pindolol 5 mg Step 2: β-blocker group received diuretics; diuretics group received a β-blocker	Significant reduction in all-cause mortality (43%), CV events (40%) and strokes (47%).
Syst-Eur (1997)	4695	Age: >60 years (mean 70.3) BP 160-219/<95 mmHg	SBP <150 mmHg	Step 1: Nitrendipine 10-40 mg daily Step 2: Enalapril 5-20 mg daily and/or HCTZ 12.5-25 mg daily	Significant reduction in CV events (31%) and strokes (42%) but no reduction in all-cause mortality.
Syst-China (1998)	2394	Mean age: 66.5 years	No targets	Step 1: Nitrendipine 10-40 mg daily Step 2: Captopril 12.5-50.0 mg daily and/or HCTZ 12.5-50.0 mg daily	Significant reduction in strokes by 38%, all-cause mortality by 39%, CV mortality by 39%, stroke mortality by 58% and all fatal and nonfatal CV endpoints by 37%.
HYVET (2008)	3845	Age: 80-105 years (mean 84.0) SBP 160-199 mmHg	BP <150/80 mmHg	Step 1: Indapamide SR 1.5 mg daily Step 2: Perindopril 2-4 mg daily	Significant reduction in CV events (34%), all-cause mortality (21%) and fatal strokes (39%).

BP: Blood pressure, CV: Cardiovascular; DBP: Diastolic blood pressure, HCTZ: Hydrochlorothiazide, SBP: Systolic blood pressure, SR: Slow release.

The Hypertension in the Very Elderly Trial (HYVET) randomized 3845 patients aged 80 years and above with SBP ≥160 mmHg to antihypertensive therapy or double-blind placebo [14]. The target BP was 150/80 mmHg. After a median follow-up of 1.8 years, participants in the antihypertensive group had a 21% reduction in all-cause mortality, a 30% reduction in fatal or nonfatal stroke, a 23% reduction in CV death and a 64% reduction in heart failure [14]. The NNT over 2.1 years to prevent one death is 46 patients. The study was terminated early because a statistically significant reduction in all-cause mortality in the active group was achieved. An important consideration of the HYVET study is that the study population was healthier than the typical older patients. For example, in HYVET, 12% of participants had a history of CV disease compared with 20.8% of women and 35.5% of men aged 80 years and above in the US [4].

The Systolic Hypertension in Europe (Syst-Eur) study randomized 4695 patients with a mean age of 70.3 years with isolated systolic hypertension to antihypertensive therapy or placebo [18]. Participants were followed up for a median of 2 years. Mean reduction in BP of 23/7 mmHg was observed in the drug therapy group compared to 13/2 mmHg in the placebo group. All-cause mortality was not significantly reduced but fatal and nonfatal strokes were reduced by 42% [18]. Fatal and nonfatal CV events were reduced by 31% [18].

Another study on systolic hypertension in China (Syst-China) alternately assigned 2394 participants with a mean age of 66.5 years to antihypertensive therapy or placebo [19]. After a mean follow-up period of 3 years, BP was reduced by 10.9/1.9 mmHg in the placebo group compared to 20.0/5.0 mmHg in the drug therapy group. In the drug therapy group, all-cause mortality was reduced by 39%, all strokes by 38%, CV mortality by 39% and stroke mortality by 58% [19].

MANAGEMENT – LIFESTYLE MODIFICATIONS

Lifestyle measures should be encouraged both to prevent the onset of hypertension and as an adjunct intervention in those with hypertension. In a meta-analysis of 56 randomized controlled trials, a mean BP reduction of 3.7/0.9 mmHg can be achieved in older hypertensive individuals with a reduction of 100 mmol/day in urinary sodium excretion, a proxy measure of dietary sodium intake

[20]. Current guidelines recommend no more than 2300 mg of sodium (or 6 g of sodium chloride daily) to no more than 1500 mg of sodium daily in older people, or those with hypertension, diabetes mellitus and chronic kidney disease [1]. In a study of 1981 Taiwanese veterans with a mean age of 75 years, participants were randomized to a regular salt diet or to a potassium-enriched salt diet with 50% less sodium [21]. Follow-up at 31 months found CV mortality to be reduced by 41% in the group receiving potassium-enriched and sodium-reduced diet.

In addition to dietary sodium restriction, adopting the Dietary Approaches to Stop Hypertension, known as the DASH eating plan (diet rich in fruits, vegetables and low-fat dairy products but low in saturated and total fat), increased physical activity and moderation of alcohol intake (less than the equivalent of two standard drinks per day for men and one for women) have been shown to reduce BP and improve other CV risk factors [22].

MANAGEMENT – PHARMACOLOGICAL TREATMENT

The five main classes of antihypertensive drugs that may be used as initial therapy for primary hypertension in older people are angiotensin-converting enzyme (ACE) inhibitors, angiotensin receptor blockers (ARBs), beta-blockers, calcium channel antagonists, and diuretics. A meta-analysis of 147 randomized trials including 464,000 adults with hypertension revealed that all five classes of antihypertensives have a similar reduction in acute coronary events and ischaemic strokes for a given decrease in BP [23]. Regardless of pre-treatment BP and the presence or absence of previous CV events, the proportionate decrease in CV events was similar in this meta-analysis [23]. Extra protective effect when beta-blockers were given after myocardial infarction and a minor additional effect in preventing strokes were observed.

The selection of specific antihypertensive drugs in older people depends on efficacy, tolerability, presence of comorbidities and cost (Table **2**). For patients with hypertension and diabetes mellitus, ACE inhibitor or ARB should be included in the absence of contraindications [24]. In the setting of chronic kidney disease with or without diabetes mellitus, an ACE inhibitor or ARB should be used [25]. Beta-blockers should be used to treat older people with complex ventricular arrhythmias, heart failure after stabilization of acute symptoms, angina pectoris, previous myocardial infarction, supraventricular tachyarrhythmias such as atrial fibrillation, hyperthyroidism, preoperative hypertension or essential tremor [26]. For older patients with hypertension and heart failure, ACE inhibitors, beta-blockers and diuretics are usually used as well as aldosterone antagonists if required [27]. Calcium channel antagonists and diuretics are preferred in older patients with isolated hypertension [15].

Table 2. Choice of antihypertensives in the treatment of hypertension in the setting of coexisting medical conditions.

	ACE Inhibitors	ARBs	Beta-Blockers	Calcium Channel Antagonists[a]	Diuretics
Prior myocardial infarction or angina pectoris			+	+	
Heart failure	+	+	+		+
Rapid atrial fibrillation			+	+	
Diabetes mellitus	+	+			
Chronic kidney disease[b]	+	+			

ACE: Angiotensin-converting enzyme, ARB: Angiotensin receptor blocker

[a]Non-dihydropyridine

[b]With or without diabetes mellitus

The choice of antihypertensive drug to use in older people is not well studied. Older people often have coexisting medical conditions, are taking multiple medications and are more prone to drug interactions which may limit the ability to achieve BP targets [28].

MANAGEMENT OF RESISTANT HYPERTENSION

Data from retrospective cross-sectional population studies of BP control in Spain and the US indicate prevalence of resistant hypertension was 7.6-8.9% [29, 30]. Post-hoc analysis of data from large clinical trials of antihypertensive therapy such as ALLHAT, ASCOT and ACCOMPLISH indicate that the prevalence could be as high as 35% [31 - 33]. Before the diagnosis of resistant hypertension is made, pseudo-resistant hypertension must be excluded. Pseudo-resistant hypertension may arise from incorrect BP measurement technique, the "white-coat" effect, lack of patient adherence to prescribed treatment or suboptimal antihypertensive therapy.

Resistant hypertension can be caused by potentially remediable secondary aetiologies such as renal artery stenosis, chronic kidney disease (either as the cause or consequence of chronic poorly-controlled hypertension), hyperaldosteronism and obstructive sleep apnoea (Table **3**).

Table 3. Common secondary causes of resistant hypertension and their relevant features.

Secondary Cause	**Features**
Renal artery stenosis	Carotid, renal or femoral bruits, flash pulmonary oedema, young females (fibromuscular dysplasia), history of atherosclerotic disease
Renal parenchymal disease	Albuminuria/proteinuria, microscopic haematuria, biochemical disturbances, peripheral oedema
Primary hyperaldosteronism	Hypokalaemia, low renin levels despite taking medications that would be expected to raise renin levels, raised aldosterone levels
Obstructive sleep apnoea	Obesity, short neck, daytime sleepiness, snoring, frequent night-time awakenings, witnessed apnoea

In older patients with resistant hypertension despite use of three different classes of antihypertensive agents, some data support the use of spironolactone as a fourth drug if the potassium is ≤4.5 mmol/L [34]. Spironolactone inhibits the action of aldosterone at the mineralocorticoid receptor, which results in natriuresis and reduction of fluid overload. The main long-term adverse effect of spironolactone is breast tenderness and gynaecomastia. It is usually reversible when the drug is stopped. Hyperkalaemia is a risk when using spironolactone in patients with resistant hypertension who are already taking an ACE inhibitor or ARB especially in those with chronic kidney disease or diabetes mellitus [35]. Therefore potassium concentration should be checked within two weeks of drug initiation and further monitoring depending on index result and dose adjustment. Hyponatraemia may also develop with long-term use, especially in older patients and when used in combination with pre-existing diuretic therapy [35]. Centrally acting α agonist such as methyldopa or vasodilators like hydralazine or minoxidil are further options.

There is growing interest in the use of devices to manage resistant hypertension so that BP control can be achieved without adding more medications. Two techniques are being assessed: percutaneous transluminal radiofrequency sympathetic denervation of the renal artery [36 - 38] and carotid baroreflex activation [39]. The Symplicity HTN-1 and HTN-2 trials have demonstrated significant BP decline in response to renal denervation, in the magnitude of 30/15 mmHg and maintained beyond two years of extended follow-up [36, 38]. These participants continued to require antihypertensive therapy but at a reduced number or dose in some patients. However, the Symplicity HTN-3 study has shown that the renal denervation group and the sham-group had similar reductions in BP [37, 40]. In older people with resistant hypertension, renal denervation has not been found to be more effective than a sham operation in reducing BP [37, 40].

CHALLENGES OF HYPERTENSION MANAGEMENT IN OLDER PEOPLE

Older people are undertreated for hypertension [1]. Medical professionals must recognise that "clinical inertia" is an important contributor to the inadequate management of hypertension in older people especially when patients require multiple antihypertensive medications. This clinical inertia can encompass a lack of knowledge about clinical guidelines, a misguided acceptance of high BP measurements or an underestimation of CV diseases risk, resulting in suboptimal treatment of hypertension [41].

While the benefit for intensive BP control has been validated in older people between the age of 65 and 80 years, evidence is lacking for the older patients, those aged above 80 years. There is a paucity of data to direct therapy in the population aged >80 years along with concerns raised by epidemiological studies regarding BP targets [42, 43].

Postural hypotension should be evaluated in all older people on antihypertensive treatment by measuring their BP with them standing for 1-3 min. Postural hypotension is defined as a drop in SBP of ≥20 mmHg or DBP of ≥10 mmHg within 3 min of standing. In a study of long-term residents of a health care facility, postural hypotension occurred in 13% of patients receiving CV or psychotropic drugs compared to 3% ($p < 0.001$) in those not receiving these drugs

[44]. Of major concerns, postural hypotension can lead to syncope, falls and potentially fractures.

Although low-dose diuretic was found to be beneficial in the HYVET study, higher doses of diuretics are associated with more electrolyte disorders such as hyponatraemia which can have significant consequences in older people [35]. This can be avoided by starting diuretics at a low dose and avoiding concurrent use of medications that can also predispose to hyponatraemia.

Poor adherence to antihypertensive therapy in the older population is another important consideration in BP control. As a result careful monitoring of adherence is essential in optimizing hypertension management. Factors that adversely affect adherence to treatment include patients' low level of education, the presence of coexisting diseases and complex medication regimens [45].

CONCLUSION

Our population is aging, and as most elderly people (≥65 years of age) are affected by hypertension, these individuals are more likely to have organ damage or clinical CVD. They major management dilemmas because most hypertension trials had upper age limits during recruitment or did not present age-specific results. Because the lack of information for evidence-based guidelines to manage older patients with hypertension, recommendations in this chapter are based on expert opinion which still provides a reasonable clinical approach. Drug treatment for elderly hypertensive patients has been generally recommended but with a greater degree of caution due to alterations in drug pharmacokinetics and pharmacodynamics with increasing age. Within the limitations of individual patient characteristics such as limited life expectancy, adverse effects of medications and coexisting diseases, treatment of hypertension is still generally beneficial among older people.

CONFLICT OF INTEREST

The author confirms that author has no conflict of interest to declare for this publication.

ACKNOWLEDGEMENTS

Declared none.

KEY POINTS

- Hypertension commonly affects older people (>65 years of age).
- Strong evidence that better blood pressure control reduces cardiovascular diseases and stroke in older people in the age group of 65-80 years.
- Evidence that tight blood pressure control in those aged 80 years or above significantly reduces cardiovascular diseases and stroke is not as strong.
- The choice of specific antihypertensive drugs in older people depends on efficacy, tolerability, presence of comorbidities and cost.
- Challenges in management of hypertension in older people may include clinical inertia, polypharmacy, coexisting diseases and postural hypotension.

REFERENCES

[1] Aronow WS, Fleg JL, Pepine CJ, *et al.* ACCF/AHA 2011 expert consensus document on hypertension in the elderly: a report of the American College of Cardiology Foundation Task Force on Clinical Expert Consensus documents developed in collaboration with the American Academy of Neurology, American Geriatrics Society, American Society for Preventive Cardiology, American Society of Hypertension, American Society of Nephrology, Association of Black Cardiologists, and European Society of Hypertension. J Am Coll Cardiol 2011; 57(20): 2037-114. [http://dx.doi.org/10.1016/j.jacc.2011.01.008] [PMID: 21524875]

[2] Calhoun DA, Jones D, Textor S, *et al.* Resistant hypertension: diagnosis, evaluation, and treatment. A scientific statement from the American Heart Association Professional Education Committee of the Council for High Blood Pressure Research. Hypertension 2008; 51(6): 1403-19. [http://dx.doi.org/10.1161/HYPERTENSIONAHA.108.189141] [PMID: 18391085]

[3] Burt VL, Whelton P, Roccella EJ, *et al.* Prevalence of hypertension in the US adult population. Results from the Third National Health and Nutrition Examination Survey, 1988-1991. Hypertension 1995; 25(3): 305-13. [http://dx.doi.org/10.1161/01.HYP.25.3.305] [PMID: 7875754]

[4] Lloyd-Jones D, Adams R, Carnethon M, *et al.* Heart disease and stroke statistics--2009 update: a report from the American Heart Association Statistics Committee and Stroke Statistics Subcommittee. Circulation 2009; 119(3): e21-e181. [http://dx.doi.org/10.1161/CIRCULATIONAHA.108.191261] [PMID: 19075105]

[5] Aronow WS, Ahmed MI, Ekundayo OJ, Allman RM, Ahmed A. A propensity-matched study of the association of peripheral arterial disease with cardiovascular outcomes in community-dwelling older adults. Am J Cardiol 2009; 103(1): 130-5. [http://dx.doi.org/10.1016/j.amjcard.2008.08.037] [PMID: 19101243]

[6] Yambe M, Tomiyama H, Yamada J, *et al.* Arterial stiffness and progression to hypertension in Japanese male subjects with high normal blood pressure. J Hypertens 2007; 25(1): 87-93. [http://dx.doi.org/10.1097/01.hjh.0000254375.73241.e2] [PMID: 17143178]

[7] Zieman SJ, Melenovsky V, Kass DA. Mechanisms, pathophysiology, and therapy of arterial stiffness. Arterioscler Thromb Vasc Biol 2005; 25(5): 932-43. [http://dx.doi.org/10.1161/01.ATV.0000160548.78317.29] [PMID: 15731494]

[8] Lind L. Systolic and diastolic hypertension impair endothelial vasodilatory function in different types of vessels in the elderly: the Prospective Investigation of the Vasculature in Uppsala Seniors (PIVUS) study. J Hypertens 2006; 24(7): 1319-27. [http://dx.doi.org/10.1097/01.hjh.0000234112.38863.6f] [PMID: 16794481]

[9] James PA, Oparil S, Carter BL, *et al.* 2014 evidence-based guideline for the management of high blood pressure in adults: report from the panel members appointed to the Eighth Joint National Committee (JNC 8). JAMA 2014; 311(5): 507-20. [http://dx.doi.org/10.1001/jama.2013.284427] [PMID: 24352797]

[10] Spence JD, Sibbald WJ, Cape RD. Pseudohypertension in the elderly. Clin Sci Mol Med Suppl 1978; 4: 399s-402s. [PMID: 282097]

[11] Prevention of stroke by antihypertensive drug treatment in older persons with isolated systolic hypertension. Final results of the Systolic Hypertension in the Elderly Program (SHEP). JAMA 1991; 265(24): 3255-64. [http://dx.doi.org/10.1001/jama.1991.03460240051027] [PMID: 2046107]

[12] Kostis JB, Davis BR, Cutler J, *et al.* Prevention of heart failure by antihypertensive drug treatment in older persons with isolated systolic hypertension. JAMA 1997; 278(3): 212-6. [http://dx.doi.org/10.1001/jama.1997.03550030052033] [PMID: 9218667]

[13] Perry HM Jr, Davis BR, Price TR, *et al.* Effect of treating isolated systolic hypertension on the risk of developing various types and subtypes of stroke: the Systolic Hypertension in the Elderly Program (SHEP). JAMA 2000; 284(4): 465-71. [http://dx.doi.org/10.1001/jama.284.4.465] [PMID: 10904510]

[14] Beckett NS, Peters R, Fletcher AE, *et al.* Treatment of hypertension in patients 80 years of age or older. N Engl J Med 2008; 358(18): 1887-98. [http://dx.doi.org/10.1056/NEJMoa0801369] [PMID: 18378519]

[15] Mancia G, Fagard R, Narkiewicz K, *et al.* 2013 ESH/ESC Guidelines for the management of arterial hypertension: the Task Force for the management of arterial hypertension of the European Society of Hypertension (ESH) and of the European Society of Cardiology (ESC). J Hypertens 2013; 31(7): 1281-357. [http://dx.doi.org/10.1097/01.hjh.0000431740.32696.cc] [PMID: 23817082]

[16] Staessen JA, Gasowski J, Wang JG, *et al.* Risks of untreated and treated isolated systolic hypertension in the elderly: meta-analysis of outcome trials. Lancet 2000; 355(9207): 865-72. [http://dx.doi.org/10.1016/S0140-6736(99)07330-4] [PMID: 10752701]

[17] Dahlöf B, Lindholm LH, Hansson L, Scherstén B, Ekbom T, Wester PO. Morbidity and mortality in

the Swedish Trial in Old Patients with Hypertension (STOP-Hypertension). Lancet 1991; 338(8778): 1281-5.
[http://dx.doi.org/10.1016/0140-6736(91)92589-T] [PMID: 1682683]

[18] Staessen JA, Fagard R, Thijs L, *et al.* Randomised double-blind comparison of placebo and active treatment for older patients with isolated systolic hypertension. Lancet 1997; 350(9080): 757-64.
[http://dx.doi.org/10.1016/S0140-6736(97)05381-6] [PMID: 9297994]

[19] Liu L, Wang JG, Gong L, Liu G, Staessen JA. Comparison of active treatment and placebo in older Chinese patients with isolated systolic hypertension. J Hypertens 1998; 16(12 Pt 1): 1823-9.
[http://dx.doi.org/10.1097/00004872-199816120-00016] [PMID: 9869017]

[20] Midgley JP, Matthew AG, Greenwood CM, Logan AG. Effect of reduced dietary sodium on blood pressure: a meta-analysis of randomized controlled trials. JAMA 1996; 275(20): 1590-7.
[http://dx.doi.org/10.1001/jama.1996.03530440070039] [PMID: 8622251]

[21] Chang HY, Hu YW, Yue CS, *et al.* Effect of potassium-enriched salt on cardiovascular mortality and medical expenses of elderly men. Am J Clin Nutr 2006; 83(6): 1289-96.
[PMID: 16762939]

[22] Appel LJ, Moore TJ, Obarzanek E, *et al.* A clinical trial of the effects of dietary patterns on blood pressure. N Engl J Med 1997; 336(16): 1117-24.
[http://dx.doi.org/10.1056/NEJM199704173361601] [PMID: 9099655]

[23] Law MR, Morris JK, Wald NJ. Use of blood pressure lowering drugs in the prevention of cardiovascular disease: meta-analysis of 147 randomised trials in the context of expectations from prospective epidemiological studies. BMJ 2009; 338: b1665.
[http://dx.doi.org/10.1136/bmj.b1665]

[24] Standards of medical care in diabetes--2013. Diabetes Care 2013; 36 (Suppl. 1): S11-66.
[http://dx.doi.org/10.2337/dc13-S011] [PMID: 23264422]

[25] Wheeler DC, Becker GJ. Summary of KDIGO guideline. What do we really know about management of blood pressure in patients with chronic kidney disease? Kidney Int 2013; 83(3): 377-83.
[http://dx.doi.org/10.1038/ki.2012.425] [PMID: 23325075]

[26] Aronow WS. Current role of beta-blockers in the treatment of hypertension. Expert Opin Pharmacother 2010; 11(16): 2599-607.
[http://dx.doi.org/10.1517/14656566.2010.482561] [PMID: 20426702]

[27] Yancy CW, Jessup M, Bozkurt B, *et al.* 2013 ACCF/AHA guideline for the management of heart failure: a report of the American College of Cardiology Foundation/American Heart Association Task Force on Practice Guidelines. J Am Coll Cardiol 2013; 62(16): e147-239.
[http://dx.doi.org/10.1016/j.jacc.2013.05.019] [PMID: 23747642]

[28] Butt TF, Branch RL, Beesley L, Martin U. Managing hypertension in the very elderly: effect of adverse drug reactions (ADRs) on achieving targets. J Hum Hypertens 2010; 24(8): 514-8.
[http://dx.doi.org/10.1038/jhh.2009.116] [PMID: 20130597]

[29] de la Sierra A, Segura J, Banegas JR, *et al.* Clinical features of 8295 patients with resistant hypertension classified on the basis of ambulatory blood pressure monitoring. Hypertension 2011; 57(5): 898-902.

[http://dx.doi.org/10.1161/HYPERTENSIONAHA.110.168948] [PMID: 21444835]

[30] Persell SD. Prevalence of resistant hypertension in the United States, 2003-2008. Hypertension 2011; 57(6): 1076-80.
[http://dx.doi.org/10.1161/HYPERTENSIONAHA.111.170308] [PMID: 21502568]

[31] Major outcomes in high-risk hypertensive patients randomized to angiotensin-converting enzyme inhibitor or calcium channel blocker vs diuretic: The Antihypertensive and Lipid-Lowering Treatment to Prevent Heart Attack Trial (ALLHAT). JAMA 2002; 288(23): 2981-97.
[http://dx.doi.org/10.1001/jama.288.23.2981] [PMID: 12479763]

[32] Gupta AK, Nasothimiou EG, Chang CL, Sever PS, Dahlöf B, Poulter NR. Baseline predictors of resistant hypertension in the Anglo-Scandinavian Cardiac Outcome Trial (ASCOT): a risk score to identify those at high-risk. J Hypertens 2011; 29(10): 2004-13.
[http://dx.doi.org/10.1097/HJH.0b013e32834a8a42] [PMID: 21881528]

[33] Jamerson K, Weber MA, Bakris GL, *et al.* Benazepril plus amlodipine or hydrochlorothiazide for hypertension in high-risk patients. N Engl J Med 2008; 359(23): 2417-28.
[http://dx.doi.org/10.1056/NEJMoa0806182] [PMID: 19052124]

[34] Chapman N, Dobson J, Wilson S, *et al.* Effect of spironolactone on blood pressure in subjects with resistant hypertension. Hypertension 2007; 49(4): 839-45.
[http://dx.doi.org/10.1161/01.HYP.0000259805.18468.8c] [PMID: 17309946]

[35] Khow KS, Lau SY, Li JY, Yong TY. Diuretic-associated electrolyte disorders in the elderly: risk factors, impact, management and prevention. Curr Drug Saf 2014; 9(1): 2-15.
[http://dx.doi.org/10.2174/1574886308666140109112730] [PMID: 24410347]

[36] Catheter-based renal sympathetic denervation for resistant hypertension: durability of blood pressure reduction out to 24 months. Hypertension 2011; 57(5): 911-7.
[http://dx.doi.org/10.1161/HYPERTENSIONAHA.110.163014] [PMID: 21403086]

[37] Bhatt DL, Kandzari DE, O'Neill WW, *et al.* A controlled trial of renal denervation for resistant hypertension. N Engl J Med 2014; 370(15): 1393-401.
[http://dx.doi.org/10.1056/NEJMoa1402670] [PMID: 24678939]

[38] Esler MD, Krum H, Schlaich M, Schmieder RE, Böhm M, Sobotka PA. Renal sympathetic denervation for treatment of drug-resistant hypertension: one-year results from the Symplicity HTN-2 randomized, controlled trial. Circulation 2012; 126(25): 2976-82.
[http://dx.doi.org/10.1161/CIRCULATIONAHA.112.130880] [PMID: 23248063]

[39] Alnima T, Kroon AA, de Leeuw PW. Baroreflex activation therapy for patients with drug-resistant hypertension. Expert Rev Cardiovasc Ther 2014; 12(8): 955-62.
[http://dx.doi.org/10.1586/14779072.2014.931226] [PMID: 25017430]

[40] Bakris GL, Townsend RR, Liu M, *et al.* Impact of renal denervation on 24-hour ambulatory blood pressure: results from SYMPLICITY HTN-3. J Am Coll Cardiol 2014; 64(11): 1071-8.
[http://dx.doi.org/10.1016/j.jacc.2014.05.012] [PMID: 24858423]

[41] Oliveria SA, Lapuerta P, McCarthy BD, L'Italien GJ, Berlowitz DR, Asch SM. Physician-related barriers to the effective management of uncontrolled hypertension. Arch Intern Med 2002; 162(4): 413-20.

[http://dx.doi.org/10.1001/archinte.162.4.413] [PMID: 11863473]

[42] Lagaay AM, van Asperen IA, Hijmans W. The prevalence of morbidity in the oldest old, aged 85 and over: a population-based survey in Leiden, The Netherlands. Arch Gerontol Geriatr 1992; 15(2): 115-31.
[http://dx.doi.org/10.1016/0167-4943(92)90012-S] [PMID: 15374369]

[43] Rastas S, Pirttilä T, Viramo P, *et al.* Association between blood pressure and survival over 9 years in a general population aged 85 and older. J Am Geriatr Soc 2006; 54(6): 912-8.
[http://dx.doi.org/10.1111/j.1532-5415.2006.00742.x] [PMID: 16776785]

[44] Aronow WS, Lee NH, Sales FF, Etienne F. Prevalence of postural hypotension in elderly patients in a long-term health care facility. Am J Cardiol 1988; 62(4): 336.
[http://dx.doi.org/10.1016/0002-9149(88)90243-3] [PMID: 3135742]

[45] Wang W, Lau Y, Loo A, Chow A, Thompson DR. Medication adherence and its associated factors among Chinese community-dwelling older adults with hypertension. Heart Lung 2014; 43(4): 278-83.
[http://dx.doi.org/10.1016/j.hrtlng.2014.05.001] [PMID: 24856232]

CHAPTER 4

Crossing New Frontiers in the Care of Older Adults with Diabetes Mellitus

Tuck Yean Yong[1,*], Kareeann Sok Fun Khow[2]

[1] *Internal Medicine, Flinders Private Hospital, Flinders Drive, Bedford Park, South Australia 5042, Australia*

[2] *Aged and Extended Care Services, The Queen Elizabeth Hospital and Department of Medicine, University of Adelaide, Adelaide, South Australia, Australia*

Abstract: Diabetes mellitus has a significant impact on the health and well-being of older people with this condition. The prevalence of diabetes and its associated complications is increasing in older people, leading to decline in functional status and quality of life. The appropriateness of tight glycaemic, blood pressure and lipid control for an older person with diabetes needs to be assessed individually. Although many pharmacological treatments for diabetes are available, their use in older people can be challenging due to increased risk of adverse reactions and drug-drug interactions with other medications. Rates of geriatric syndromes (*e.g.* depression, cognitive impairment, functional disability, urinary incontinence and falls) are increased in older people with diabetes. Multidisciplinary and multidimensional approach to management is essential to maintain independence and quality of life in older people with diabetes.

Keywords: Cardiovascular diseases, Diabetes mellitus, Geriatric syndromes, Glycated haemoglobin, Hyperglycaemia, Hypertension, Hypoglycaemia, Individualized therapy, Older people.

INTRODUCTION

Diabetes mellitus is more common in the older population. More than 20% of the US population aged ≥65 years has diabetes [1] and the ageing population is a

* **Correspondence author Tuck Yean Yong**: Internal Medicine, Flinders Private Hospital, Flinders Drive, Bedford Park, South Australia 5042, Australia; Tel: +61 8 8241 2121; Fax: +61 8 8240 0879; E-mail: tyyong@hotmail.com.

significant driver of the diabetes epidemic. Similarly in China, the prevalence of diabetes in the population aged 60 years and above was about 20% [2]. Older people with diabetes may either have newly diagnosed disease (diagnosed after 65 years of age) or long-standing diagnosis with onset before 65 years of age. Older people with diabetes have type 2 diabetes (>90%) and 75% of them are estimated to require insulin therapy [3]. The burden of diabetes in older people is associated with higher mortality, reduced functional status and increased risk of institutionalization [4]. Older adults with diabetes are also at higher risk for both acute and chronic cardiovascular and microvascular complications related to this disease.

The treatment of diabetes in the older population, especially the older old (aged ≥80 years), is often challenging because therapy options are limited by their physical, psychological and cognitive functions. Older patients with diabetes may have increased risk for frailty and functional dependency [5]. Although there is currently no gold standard definition of frailty, it is generally considered to be a multi-factorial condition characterised by a heightened vulnerability to changes in health status [6]. This chapter will focus on the features of diabetes relevant to older people, currently available treatment options, geriatric syndromes in the setting of diabetes and challenges of management in this age group.

PATHOGENESIS

Older people are at higher risk for developing type 2 diabetes because insulin resistance increases and pancreatic islet function declines with increasing age. Age-related insulin resistance has been found to be associated with adiposity, sarcopenia and physical inactivity [7]. In addition, age-related deterioration in pancreatic islet function and islet proliferation have also been reported [8 - 10].

Insulin secretion has been observed to decline with age, with considerably diminished β-cell sensitivity and acute insulin response [11]. In contrast to younger people, insulin resistance in older people with type 2 diabetes seems to predominate in skeletal muscle, whereas hepatic glucose output is almost unaffected [11]. One of the most striking changes in older people with type 2 diabetes is the presence of insulin resistance in the absence of obesity, which could be linked to mitochondrial dysfunction in skeletal muscle and increased fat accumulation in muscle and liver tissue [12, 13]. Type 2 diabetes in older lean people is usually associated with a significant impairment in glucose-induced insulin secretion, whereas in older obese people, the main deficit seems to be resistance to insulin-mediated glucose disposal [13, 14].

SCREENING AND DIAGNOSIS

Clinical presentation of diabetes in old age is often non-specific and asymptomatic resulting in delay in diagnosis. In general, screening and diagnosis of diabetes in older subjects should be in accordance with published international or national criteria and guidelines [15, 16]. Currently no age-defined criteria has been proposed. Frequent healthcare contact for other medical problems in the absence of diabetes-related symptoms may reveal incidental cases of diabetes. For example type 2 diabetes in older people can present as falls, urinary incontinence and changes in cognition or behaviour.

Three important factors have been identified that increase the value of screening for diabetes: age ≥55 years, systolic blood pressure of ≥130 mmHg, or a body mass index ≥35 kg/m^2 [17]. However no agreement exists on the best screening test for diabetes in people aged ≥55 years. When fasting plasma glucose is the only criterion used, the prevalence and incidence rates of diabetes in older people (>65 years) may be underestimated [18]. In higher-risk older people with a normal fasting glucose where an oral glucose tolerance test (OGTT) is not feasible, determination of glycated haemoglobin (HbA_{1c}) may be helpful in the diagnosis of diabetes [19]. An HbA_{1c} 48 mmol/mol or >6.5% may indicate the likely presence of diabetes [19].

ASSESSMENT

Older patients with type 2 diabetes should have an evaluation of their overall functional status using well-validated assessment tools [20]. Incorporating a comprehensive geriatric assessment will ensure the assessment of three major domains: global/physical, cognitive and affective [20]. In older adults with diabetes, functional status can dictate the screening, preventive, diagnostic and therapeutic approach, including therapeutic targets.

DIABETES CARE IN OLDER PEOPLE

Current clinical practice in glycaemic control in type 2 diabetes is largely influenced by the findings of several multi-centre clinical studies namely the UK Prospective Diabetes Study (UKPDS), the Action to Control Cardiovascular Risk in Diabetes (ACCORD), the Action in Diabetes and Vascular Disease: Preterax and Diamicron MR Controlled Evaluation (ADVANCE) and the Veterans Affairs Diabetes Trial (VADT) [21 - 25]. The UKPDS provided evidence that intensive glycaemic control is beneficial for reducing the risk of microvascular complications but this study excluded patients aged ≥65 years at the time of enrolment [21, 22]. The ACCORD trial was terminated after about 3 years because of excessive deaths in the intensive glucose control group [23]. The ADVANCE trial showed there was significant reduction in the incidence of nephropathy but not cardiovascular events or death [24]. Like ADVANCE, VADT also did not reveal any significant effect of intensive glucose control on major cardiovascular events or deaths [25]. ACCORD, ADVANCE and VADT trials have caused uncertainties regarding the benefits and risks of intensive glycaemic therapy in older people.

For independent or robust older patients with type 2 diabetes, with single system involvement and no other major comorbidities, attaining target HbA_{1c} of 53-58 mmol/mol (7.0-7.5%) is desirable (Table **1**) [26]. However the exact target in individual patients will depend on existing cardiovascular risk, presence of microvascular complications and ability to self-manage glycaemic therapies. For frail patients such as those who are dependent, residents of aged care facilities, have multisystem diseases or dementia, the risk of hypoglycaemia is high and the aim of therapy should be symptom control and prevention of metabolic decompensation. Generally the target HbA_{1c} of 60-69 mmol/mol (7.6-8.5%) and/or fasting glucose of 7.6-9.0 mmol/L is reasonable [26].

The benefits of intensive blood pressure control in older people with type 2 diabetes has been extrapolated from studies of older adults with hypertension but not restricted to those with diabetes [27]. There is consistent evidence that reducing blood pressure from very high levels (≥170 mmHg) to moderate targets (such as 150 mmHg) reduces cardiovascular events in older people with diabetes

[28]. However, data is lacking on the benefits of achieving lower blood pressure targets (systolic blood pressure <120 mmHg or diastolic blood pressure <70 mmHg) [29].

Table 1. Suggested therapeutic targets for cardiovascular risk factors according to functional status of older people with type 2 diabetes.

	Independent or Robust	**Frail or Mild Disability**	**Moderate-to-Severe Disability**	**End of Life**
HbA1c	53-59 mmol/mol (7.0-7.5%)	53-64 mmol/mol (7.0-8.0%)	<69 mmol/mol (<8.5%)	Avoid symptomatic hypoglycaemia
Blood pressure	<140/90 mmHg	<140/90 mmHg	<150/90 mmHg	Avoid short-term life-threatening elevated blood pressure
LDL cholesterol	<2.0 mmol/L (individualised in aged ≥80 years)	Individualise	Not necessary	Not necessary
HDL cholesterol	>1.0 mmol/L	Individualise	Not necessary	Not necessary

No large interventional trials for lipid-lowering involving only older people with diabetes have been reported. As a result, benefits of lipid-lowering therapy in the older population with diabetes have been inferred from either studies of older adults which included those with diabetes or those with diabetes that included older people. A meta-analysis of 18,686 people with diabetes in 14 trials using statin therapy for primary prevention found a 20% relative reduction in major adverse vascular events in those over the age of 65 years [30]. For secondary prevention of cardiovascular disease, statin trials in adults with diabetes have found relative reductions in recurrent cardiovascular events and mortality by age group [27]. However, subgroup analyses of the Fenofibrate Intervention and Event Lowering in Diabetes (FIELD) study, which showed some benefit of this medication in people with type 2 diabetes, did not demonstrate any benefit for those aged ≥65 years [31].

Non-Pharmacological Interventions

Physical activity and addressing nutritional issues are an integral part of diabetes care for all ages. In older people with diabetes, muscle mass and strength decline with age, and these deterioration may be exacerbated by diabetes complications, comorbidities and recurrent hospitalizations. Adults with diabetes of longer duration and/or higher HbA_{1c} have lower muscle strength per unit of muscle mass than BMI- and age-matched people with diabetes and those with a shorter duration of disease or better glycaemic control [32]. Therefore physical activity interventions to improve the functional status of older people with or without diabetes are vital [33]. In the Look AHEAD (Action for Health in Diabetes) study, subjects aged 65-76 years had improved gains in fitness after intensive lifestyle intervention [34]. In older adults, even light-intensity physical activity is associated with higher self-rated physical health and psychosocial wellbeing [35].

Although energy requirements decline with age, macronutrient needs are similar throughout adulthood [36]. Meeting micronutrient needs is more challenging in older people because of reduced caloric intake and the elderly with diabetes are at higher risk of deficiencies [37]. Furthermore older people are at increased risk of malnutrition because of anorexia of ageing, altered taste and smell, swallowing difficulties, dental or oral issues and functional impairments leading to lack of ability to prepare food [38]. Therefore overly restrictive pattern, whether provider-directed or self-imposed, should be avoided in older people with diabetes.

Obesity and overweight are prevalent among older adults with diabetes. Obesity can be associated with sarcopenia [39]. Obesity also exacerbates the decline in physical function and increases the risk of frailty [40]. While unintentional weight loss is a known nutritional concern, intentional weight loss in obese and overweight older adults could potentially worsen sarcopenia, bone mineral density and nutritional deficits [41, 42]. Therefore strategies that combine physical activity with nutritional interventions to promote weight loss may be more beneficial in improving physical function and cardiometabolic risk profile in older people [40, 41].

Pharmacological Interventions for Glycaemic Control

Older patients are at increased risk for adverse drug events because of age-related changes in pharmacokinetics (especially reduced renal drug clearance) and pharmacodynamics (increased sensitivity with certain medications). These changes can lead to increased risk of hypoglycaemia, the potential need to reduce doses of some medications and attention to kidney function [43, 44]. Furthermore polypharmacy (usually more than five regular medications per person), medication burden, high cost and lack of adherence compound pharmacological interventions in older people. In general there is a lack of comparison effectiveness studies on medications used for glycaemic control in older people with type 2 diabetes.

Metformin is often considered the first-line treatment for type 2 diabetes because it has a low risk of hypoglycaemia. However gastrointestinal adverse effects and weight loss with the use of this drug can be a problem in frail patients. Lactic acidosis with metformin use is rare (incidence of 9 in 100,00 person years) [45] and increasing age is not a risk factor. However lactic acidosis is of greater concern in patients using metformin with advanced kidney impairment, exposure to iodinated contrast agents and clinical situations with reduced tissue perfusion. Therefore the dose of metformin should be reduced if the estimated glomerular filtration rate (eGFR) is 30-60 mL/min/1.73 m^2 (Table **2**) [46]. Metformin should be avoided if eGFR is $<$30 mL/min/1.73 m^2 [47]. A potential benefit of metformin may include slowing the loss of muscle mass in older men with diabetes [48].

Sulphonylureas are effective both as monotherapy and in combination with other agents that have different mechanisms. This class of drug can lower the HbA_{1c} by 11-22 mmol/mol (1-2%) as monotherapy [49]. Sulphonylureas have been considered as a first-line therapy in lean older people with diabetes [49]. However sulphonylureas are associated with weight gain and increased risk of hypoglycaemia. In particular, glibenclamide or glyburide is associated with a higher risk of hypoglycaemia in older people and should be avoided in this age group [50]. Gliclazide, glipizide and glimepiride are sulphonylureas that can be used in older people. This group of medications should be used cautiously in the presence of hepatic and renal impairment because the primary site of metabolism and elimination are the liver and kidneys, respectively (Table **2**).

Thiazolidinediones can be effective for glycaemic control in older people with a dose-dependent glycaemic-lowering effect (HbA_{1c} reduction of about 15 mmol/mol or 1.5%) [49]. This class of drug rarely cause hypoglycaemia unless used in conjunction with sulphonylureas or insulin. Thiazolidinediones have been used in older people with obesity, those with contraindications or intolerance to metformin, or as an adjunct therapy in those who have inadequate glycaemic control despite high insulin requirements. However in older people, the incidence of anaemia and oedema is higher in older people treated with thiazolidinediones [51]. Therefore, volume status and blood count have to be monitored closely. Furthermore, older people on rosiglitazone have a higher risk of cardiovascular morbidity and mortality [52].

Like sulphonylureas, meglitinides stimulate insulin secretion from the β cell and can reduce HbA_{1c} by 11-22 mmol/mol (1-2%) [49]. However these agents have a rapid onset and very short duration of action [53]. In older people, nateglinide monotherapy or in combination with metformin produces significant improvements in glycaemic control and is well tolerated [54]. Meglitinides may be an option for older people who have irregular eating patterns and have frequent hypoglycaemia while taking sulfonylureas. These advantages need to be balanced against the cost and adherence, especially among patients with cognitive impairment and polypharmacy [55].

α-Glucosidase inhibitors such as acarbose can improve postprandial hyperglycaemia and have a modest reduction of HbA_{1c} by 5-11 mmol/mol (0.5-1.0%) [56]. In a small study of older people (≥65 years of age), the efficacy of acarbose can be achieved at a low dose of 25 mg before each meal but the adverse effects of this class of medication have a greater negative effect on older people with poor mobility, where functional bowel incontinence may occur [57].

Dipeptidyl peptidase-4 (DPP-4) inhibitors have been shown to improve glycaemic control in older people (aged ≥65 years) with a reduction of HbA_{1c} of 5-8 mmol/mol (0.5-0.8%) [58 - 62]. This medication class is also tolerated well and is associated with minimal risk of hypoglycaemia [63]. In patients with renal impairment, dose adjustment of sitagliptin, saxagliptin, vildagliptin and alogliptin is required but not for linagliptin. However data on the long-term safety, tolerability, durability and cost-effectiveness of DPP-4 inhibitors in different subgroups of older people with diabetes, are still needed.

Glucagon-like peptide-1 receptor (GLP-1) agonists can lead to moderate reductions of HbA_{1c} of 5-11 mmol/mol (0.5-1.0%) in older people with diabetes by enhancing glucose-induced insulin release and increase insulin sensitivity [64, 65]. They may be indicated as an adjunct therapy for glycaemic management in people who are not achieving adequate control with other oral agents or basal insulin. However injection therapy may add to regimen complexity and its high cost may be a hindrance. In addition, long-term data is still lacking on benefits, safety and tolerability of these agents in older people with diabetes.

Table 2. Dose adjustments of selective hypoglycaemic agents in the setting of deteriorating kidney function.

	Stages of Chronic Kidney Disease (Based on eGFR, mL/min/1.73 m2)			
	Stages 1 and 2 (> 60)	Stages 3A and 3B (30-60)	Stage 4 (15-30)	Stage 5 (<15/dialysis)
Metformin		DR	Avoid	Avoid
Acarbose			Avoid	Avoid
Linagliptin				
Sitagliptin		DR	DR	DR
Saxagliptin		DR	DR	Avoid
Vildagliptin		DR	DR	Avoid
Dapagliflozin			Avoid	Avoid

Shaded boxes indicate no dosage adjustment is required.
DR: Dose reduction, eGFR: estimated glomerular filtration rate

Sodium glucose cotransporter 2 (SGLT-2) inhibitors reduce glucose reabsorption at the proximal tubule, increasing urinary excretion and thereby leads to a reduction in plasma glucose concentration. The use of SGLT-2 inhibitors is associated with HbA1c reduction of 7-11 mmol/mol (0.7-1.0%) [66, 67]. Canaglifloxin has been shown to improve glycaemic control, reduce systolic blood pressure and body weight, and generally tolerated well by older people with type 2 diabetes [66]. One study has also shown efficacy and safety of use in older people with concurrent diabetes and chronic kidney disease [67]. However, urinary tract infection and osmotic-related adverse events can be barriers to their use in frail older people [66]. In addition, these agents are still relatively new in clinical use and there is more to learn about its role in glycaemic treatment of older people.

Amylin analogues such as pramlintide are a synthetic analogue of human amylin which can be used as an adjunct to insulin because of its ability to enhance the effects of insulin [68]. Pramlintinde decreases HbA_{1c} by 3 mmol/mol (0.3%) and may also lead to some weight loss [68]. It is approved for use in the USA but it may not be available in other countries. This agent should be used with caution in older people because of high risk of hypoglycaemia and requires two or three injections each day [68]. It is not a suitable option for older people with cognitive, visual or functional impairment and high risk of hypoglycaemia.

Generally as diabetes progresses, the maximum dose of non-insulin agents is unable to maintain glucose control at personalized targets and insulin is required. In one study of healthy and functional older people (mean age of 66 years), mean HbA_{1c} of 53 mmol/mol (7.0%) was achieved and maintained for 12 months with low rates of hypoglycaemia through either an insulin subcutaneous infusion or multiple daily injections [69]. Similarly, the addition of long-acting insulin was effective in achieving HbA_{1c} goals for older people with type 2 diabetes (mean age of 69 years) in a number of trials [48]. However limited data is available about insulin therapy in people over the age of 75 years or those with multiple comorbidities and/or limited functional status. Functional, visual, psychological and cognitive impairments may limit the efficacy and safety of the use of insulin in some older people. As diabetes progresses, health care providers have to balance the complexity of the insulin regimen, the personalized glucose target and the actual ability of older adults or their support system, to implement such a regimen.

DIABETES AND GERIATRIC SYNDROMES

Diabetes is associated with increased incidence of geriatric syndromes such as frailty, depression, cognitive impairment, urinary incontinence, functional disability and falls. Hyperglycaemia and diabetes-related micro- and macrovascular complications are contributing factors to geriatric syndromes. On the other hand, geriatric syndromes have a significant influence on the treatment and care of older people with diabetes.

Diabetes significantly increases the risk of frailty [70]. Furthermore, macrovascular complications are powerful predictors of progression of frailty in older people with diabetes [71]. Frailty has a high predictive power for adverse outcomes in older adults, including disability, admission to hospital, permanent institutionalization, falls and death [6].

About 30% of people with diabetes have symptoms of depression and 5-10% have features meeting the criteria for major depression [72]. Untreated depression can lead to difficulties with self-care and implementation of healthy lifestyle choices [73]. The presence of untreated depression is also associated with a higher risk of mortality, disability and macro- and microvascular complications in older patients with type 2 diabetes [74]. Clinical tools such as the Geriatric Depression Scale can be used in the initial assessment of older people with diabetes [75]. A combination of psychological interventions (counselling, group therapy and cognitive behavioural therapy) and antidepressants (such as selective serotonin-reuptake inhibitors) may be necessary for the treatment of depression in older people with diabetes [76].

Epidemiological studies have shown that people with diabetes have a 1.6-2.0-fold increased risk for Alzheimer's and vascular dementia [77, 78]. Hyperglycaemia, advanced glycated end products, recurrent severe hypoglycaemia, asymptomatic and symptomatic cerebrovascular disease and insulin resistance have been found to be associated with cognitive decline in diabetes [79 - 83]. Although patients with diabetes, treated with insulin, had a higher risk of cognitive impairment or dementia, the association may be because of increased cerebral complications rather than the effects of insulin [77, 79]. In older people with diabetes, cognitive function is an important factor influencing adherence to diabetes self-care activities, frequency of hospital admission and the need for assistance with personal care [84]. Glycaemic control in the short-term may have some favourable effects on cognitive function in people with diabetes [81, 85]. Intensive social supports are necessary for older people with diabetes and cognitive impairment to ensure treatment adherence and avoidance of complications such as hypoglycaemia.

Diabetes is associated with increased risk of both stress and urge incontinence [86 - 88]. Overflow incontinence may in older people with diabetes who develop autonomic neuropathy. In the multivariate analysis of one study, duration of diabetes, neuropathy, retinopathy and a history of urinary tract infection were independently associated with severe incontinence [87]. Useful treatment strategies for stress incontinence include pelvic floor muscle training, weight reduction and training in mobility and toileting skills [89, 90].

Functional disability is one of the most serious geriatric syndromes in older people with diabetes. Cross-sectional studies have shown that diabetes in older people was associated with a two-fold increased risk of impairment in performing daily physical tasks [91, 92]. In these studies, coronary artery disease, stroke, peripheral vascular disease, neuropathy, depression and obesity were important contributing factors to diabetes-related functional disability. Supervised muscle-strengthening training and aerobic exercise is necessary to prevent progression in disability and maintain good glycaemic control [93].

Falls, both injurious and non-injurious, adversely affect older people with diabetes. Evidence indicates that diabetes is one of the major predictors of the risk of falls [94, 95]. Studies have shown that poor lower extremity function, poor gait balance, coronary artery disease, arthritis, visual impairment, peripheral neuropathy and being overweight were associated with falling among people with diabetes [95 - 97]. As part of the annual review, older people with diabetes should have a falls risk assessment which includes identifying risk factors such as medications, environmental factors and evaluation of gait and balance. A multidisciplinary falls prevention program should be offered to all community-dwelling people with a history of a fall or at high risk of falling [98]. Current guideline also recommend that tight glycaemic control (HbA_{1c} <53 mmol/mol or 7.0%) must be avoided in older people with diabetes who are at increased risk of falling [26].

CHALLENGES IN TREATING OLDER PEOPLE WITH DIABETES

The prevalence of any hypoglycaemia (blood glucose <3.9 mmol/L or 70 mg/dL) or severe hypoglycaemia (requiring third-party assistance) among older people with diabetes is unknown. Age appears to affect counter-regulatory responses to hypoglycaemia in people without diabetes [99] but studies in those with diabetes is lacking. Assessment of risk factors for hypoglycaemia is an important part of the clinical care of older people with diabetes, especially those taking insulin or insulin secretogogues. Other strong predictors of hypoglycaemia in older people include macroalbuminuria with a long duration of type 2 diabetes, recent admission to hospital and polypharmacy [100, 101]. Risk of severe hypoglycaemia tends to be higher in people with very high HbA_{1c} (>75 mmol/mol or 9.0%) or near-normal glycaemic control (<42 mmol/mol or 6.0%), and in those with kidney insufficiency and dementia [102, 103].

Although much attention has appropriately been paid to the risks of overtreatment of hyperglycaemia in older people (treatment burden, hypoglycaemia and possible increased mortality), untreated or undertreated hyperglycaemia are associated with other risks, even for those with short life expectancy and would not be affected by chronic complications. Blood glucose levels consistently over the renal threshold for glycosuria (10.0-11.1 mmol/L or 180-200 mg/dL) increase the risks of dehydration, postural hypotension, falls, urinary incontinence and electrolyte abnormalities. Unrecognized or undertreated hyperglycaemia in older people can lead to hyperglycaemic hyperosmolar syndrome which is a severe complication. Therefore, one of the goals of diabetes treatment in older people with limited life expectancy is to minimize severe hyperglycaemia rather than tight glycaemic control.

One of the major influences on the decision-making for diabetes treatment targets or interventions in older people is life expectancy. Patients whose life expectancy is limited are considered less likely to benefit from intensive control of hyperglycaemia, blood pressure and hyperlipidaemia. However current tools are limited in predicting the life expectancy for a particular older patient with diabetes. Further research is required in this area so that treatment can be individualised in older patient with diabetes.

CONCLUSION

The management of diabetes in older people is complex and challenging.

Managing diabetes well in an older person requires an understanding of the individual's personal needs and preferences, functional, cognitive and psychological abilities, and their social environment, especially the availability, knowledge and involvement of caregivers. Although there are many pharmacological options in the management of diabetes, evidence from intervention studies in older people are still lacking, particularly data on comparative effectiveness. Future research studies on diabetes management are needed to include specific populations of older people with frailty, dementia and specialized care requirements. In older people, focus should shift from specific diabetes management to comprehensive functional assessment, individualised metabolic targeting and planning for optimum patient safety and quality.

CONFLICT OF INTEREST

The author confirms that author has no conflict of interest to declare for this publication.

ACKNOWLEDGEMENTS

Declared none.

KEY POINTS

- The prevalence of diabetes and its associated complications is increasing in older people.
- Emphasis on glycaemic control in older people should be individualized because of associated complications from overly intensive treatment.
- The pharmacological treatment of diabetes is challenging especially when interventions are associated with adverse reactions and interactions with other medications
- Diabetes in older people is associated with increased incidence of geriatric syndromes requiring careful assessment and management
- More research is needed to identify the most cost-effective and patient-centred approach to managing diabetes and associated complications in old age.

REFERENCES

[1] Cowie CC, Rust KF, Byrd-Holt DD, *et al.* Prevalence of diabetes and impaired fasting glucose in adults in the U.S. population: National Health And Nutrition Examination Survey 1999-2002. Diabetes Care 2006; 29(6): 1263-8.
[http://dx.doi.org/10.2337/dc06-0062] [PMID: 16732006]

[2] Yang W, Lu J, Weng J, *et al.* Prevalence of diabetes among men and women in China. N Engl J Med 2010; 362(12): 1090-101.
[http://dx.doi.org/10.1056/NEJMoa0908292] [PMID: 20335585]

[3] Neil HA, Thompson AV, Thorogood M, Fowler GH, Mann JI. Diabetes in the elderly: the Oxford Community Diabetes Study. Diabet Med 1989; 6(7): 608-13.
[http://dx.doi.org/10.1111/j.1464-5491.1989.tb01237.x] [PMID: 2527702]

[4] Brown AF, Mangione CM, Saliba D, Sarkisian CA. Guidelines for improving the care of the older person with diabetes mellitus. J Am Geriatr Soc 2003; 51(5) (Suppl Guidelines): S265-80.
[PMID: 12694461]

[5] Bourdel-Marchasson I, Berrut G. Caring the elderly diabetic patient with respect to concepts of successful aging and frailty. Diab Metab 2005; 31(S2): S9-S13.
[http://dx.doi.org/10.1016/S1262-3636(05)73647-8]

[6] Clegg A, Young J, Iliffe S, Rikkert MO, Rockwood K. Frailty in elderly people. Lancet 2013; 381(9868): 752-62.
[http://dx.doi.org/10.1016/S0140-6736(12)62167-9] [PMID: 23395245]

[7] Amati F, Dubé JJ, Coen PM, Stefanovic-Racic M, Toledo FG, Goodpaster BH. Physical inactivity and obesity underlie the insulin resistance of aging. Diabetes Care 2009; 32(8): 1547-9.
[http://dx.doi.org/10.2337/dc09-0267] [PMID: 19401446]

[8] Maedler K, Schumann DM, Schulthess F, *et al.* Aging correlates with decreased beta-cell proliferative capacity and enhanced sensitivity to apoptosis: a potential role for Fas and pancreatic duodenal homeobox-1. Diabetes 2006; 55(9): 2455-62.
[http://dx.doi.org/10.2337/db05-1586] [PMID: 16936193]

[9] Rankin MM, Kushner JA. Adaptive beta-cell proliferation is severely restricted with advanced age. Diabetes 2009; 58(6): 1365-72.
[http://dx.doi.org/10.2337/db08-1198] [PMID: 19265026]

[10] Reers C, Erbel S, Esposito I, *et al.* Impaired islet turnover in human donor pancreata with aging. Eur J Endocrinol 2009; 160(2): 185-91.
[http://dx.doi.org/10.1530/EJE-08-0596] [PMID: 19004984]

[11] Scheen AJ. Diabetes mellitus in the elderly: insulin resistance and/or impaired insulin secretion? Diab Metab 2005; 31: 5s27-34.

[12] Petersen KF, Befroy D, Dufour S, *et al.* Mitochondrial dysfunction in the elderly: possible role in insulin resistance. Science 2003; 300(5622): 1140-2.
[http://dx.doi.org/10.1126/science.1082889] [PMID: 12750520]

[13] Meneilly GS, Elahi D. Metabolic alterations in middle-aged and elderly lean patients with type 2 diabetes. Diabetes Care 2005; 28(6): 1498-9.

[http://dx.doi.org/10.2337/diacare.28.6.1498] [PMID: 15920078]

[14] Meneilly GS, Elliott T. Metabolic alterations in middle-aged and elderly obese patients with type 2 diabetes. Diabetes Care 1999; 22(1): 112-8. [http://dx.doi.org/10.2337/diacare.22.1.112] [PMID: 10333911]

[15] Colman PG, Thomas DW, Zimmet PZ, Welborn TA, Garcia-Webb P, Moore MP. New classification and criteria for diagnosis of diabetes mellitus. Position Statement from the Australian Diabetes Society, New Zealand Society for the Study of Diabetes, Royal College of Pathologists of Australasia and Australasian Association of Clinical Biochemists. Med J Aust 1999; 170(8): 375-8. [PMID: 10327951]

[16] Global Guideline for Type 2 Diabetes: recommendations for standard, comprehensive, and minimal care. Diabet Med 2006; 23(6): 579-93. [http://dx.doi.org/10.1111/j.1464-5491.2006.01918.x] [PMID: 16759299]

[17] Chatterjee R, Narayan KM, Lipscomb J, *et al.* Screening for diabetes and prediabetes should be cost-saving in patients at high risk. Diabetes Care 2013; 36(7): 1981-7. [http://dx.doi.org/10.2337/dc12-1752] [PMID: 23393215]

[18] Harris MI, Hadden WC, Knowler WC, Bennett PH. Prevalence of diabetes and impaired glucose tolerance and plasma glucose levels in U.S. population aged 20-74 yr. Diabetes 1987; 36(4): 523-34. [http://dx.doi.org/10.2337/diab.36.4.523] [PMID: 3817306]

[19] Motta M, Bennati E, Cardillo E, Ferlito L, Malaguarnera M. The value of glycosylated hemoglobin (HbA1c) as a predictive risk factor in the diagnosis of diabetes mellitus (DM) in the elderly. Arch Gerontol Geriatr 2010; 50(1): 60-4. [http://dx.doi.org/10.1016/j.archger.2009.01.012] [PMID: 19344959]

[20] Devons CA. Comprehensive geriatric assessment: making the most of the aging years. Curr Opin Clin Nutr Metab Care 2002; 5(1): 19-24. [http://dx.doi.org/10.1097/00075197-200201000-00004] [PMID: 11790944]

[21] Effect of intensive blood-glucose control with metformin on complications in overweight patients with type 2 diabetes (UKPDS 34). Lancet 1998; 352(9131): 854-65. [http://dx.doi.org/10.1016/S0140-6736(98)07037-8] [PMID: 9742977]

[22] Intensive blood-glucose control with sulphonylureas or insulin compared with conventional treatment and risk of complications in patients with type 2 diabetes (UKPDS 33). Lancet 1998; 352(9131): 837-53. [http://dx.doi.org/10.1016/S0140-6736(98)07019-6] [PMID: 9742976]

[23] Gerstein HC, Miller ME, Byington RP, *et al.* Effects of intensive glucose lowering in type 2 diabetes. N Engl J Med 2008; 358(24): 2545-59. [http://dx.doi.org/10.1056/NEJMoa0802743] [PMID: 18539917]

[24] Patel A, MacMahon S, Chalmers J, *et al.* Intensive blood glucose control and vascular outcomes in patients with type 2 diabetes. N Engl J Med 2008; 358(24): 2560-72. [http://dx.doi.org/10.1056/NEJMoa0802987] [PMID: 18539916]

[25] Duckworth W, Abraira C, Moritz T, *et al.* Glucose control and vascular complications in veterans with type 2 diabetes. N Engl J Med 2009; 360(2): 129-39.

[http://dx.doi.org/10.1056/NEJMoa0808431] [PMID: 19092145]

[26] Sinclair AJ, Paolisso G, Castro M, Bourdel-Marchasson I, Gadsby R, Rodriguez Mañas L. European Diabetes Working Party for Older People 2011 clinical guidelines for type 2 diabetes mellitus. Executive summary. Diabetes Metab 2011; 37 (Suppl. 3): S27-38. [http://dx.doi.org/10.1016/S1262-3636(11)70962-4] [PMID: 22183418]

[27] Cigolle CT, Blaum CS, Halter JB. Diabetes and cardiovascular disease prevention in older adults. Clin Geriatr Med 2009; 25(4): 607-641, vii-viii. [http://dx.doi.org/10.1016/j.cger.2009.09.001] [PMID: 19944264]

[28] Hansson L, Zanchetti A, Carruthers SG, *et al.* Effects of intensive blood-pressure lowering and low-dose aspirin in patients with hypertension: principal results of the Hypertension Optimal Treatment (HOT) randomised trial. Lancet 1998; 351(9118): 1755-62. [http://dx.doi.org/10.1016/S0140-6736(98)04311-6] [PMID: 9635947]

[29] Cushman WC, Evans GW, Byington RP, *et al.* Effects of intensive blood-pressure control in type 2 diabetes mellitus. N Engl J Med 2010; 362(17): 1575-85. [http://dx.doi.org/10.1056/NEJMoa1001286] [PMID: 20228401]

[30] Baigent C, Keech A, Kearney PM, *et al.* Efficacy and safety of cholesterol-lowering treatment: prospective meta-analysis of data from 90,056 participants in 14 randomised trials of statins. Lancet 2005; 366(9493): 1267-78. [http://dx.doi.org/10.1016/S0140-6736(05)67394-1] [PMID: 16214597]

[31] Keech A, Simes RJ, Barter P, *et al.* Effects of long-term fenofibrate therapy on cardiovascular events in 9795 people with type 2 diabetes mellitus (the FIELD study): randomised controlled trial. Lancet 2005; 366(9500): 1849-61. [http://dx.doi.org/10.1016/S0140-6736(05)67667-2] [PMID: 16310551]

[32] Park SW, Goodpaster BH, Strotmeyer ES, *et al.* Decreased muscle strength and quality in older adults with type 2 diabetes: the health, aging, and body composition study. Diabetes 2006; 55(6): 1813-8. [http://dx.doi.org/10.2337/db05-1183] [PMID: 16731847]

[33] Villareal DT, Chode S, Parimi N, *et al.* Weight loss, exercise, or both and physical function in obese older adults. N Engl J Med 2011; 364(13): 1218-29. [http://dx.doi.org/10.1056/NEJMoa1008234] [PMID: 21449785]

[34] Jakicic JM, Jaramillo SA, Balasubramanyam A, *et al.* Effect of a lifestyle intervention on change in cardiorespiratory fitness in adults with type 2 diabetes: results from the Look AHEAD Study. Int J Obes 2009; 33(3): 305-16. [http://dx.doi.org/10.1038/ijo.2008.280] [PMID: 19153582]

[35] Buman MP, Hekler EB, Haskell WL, *et al.* Objective light-intensity physical activity associations with rated health in older adults. Am J Epidemiol 2010; 172(10): 1155-65. [http://dx.doi.org/10.1093/aje/kwq249] [PMID: 20843864]

[36] Drewnowski A, Warren-Mears VA. Does aging change nutrition requirements? J Nutr Health Aging 2001; 5(2): 70-4. [PMID: 11426285]

[37] Elmadfa I, Meyer AL. Body composition, changing physiological functions and nutrient requirements

of the elderly. Ann Nutr Metab 2008; 52 (Suppl. 1): 2-5.
[http://dx.doi.org/10.1159/000115339] [PMID: 18382069]

[38] Visvanathan R, Chapman IM. Undernutrition and anorexia in the older person. Gastroenterol Clin North Am 2009; 38(3): 393-409.
[http://dx.doi.org/10.1016/j.gtc.2009.06.009] [PMID: 19699404]

[39] Zamboni M, Mazzali G, Fantin F, Rossi A, Di Francesco V. Sarcopenic obesity: a new category of obesity in the elderly. Nutr Metab Cardiovasc Dis 2008; 18(5): 388-95.
[http://dx.doi.org/10.1016/j.numecd.2007.10.002] [PMID: 18395429]

[40] Villareal DT, Banks M, Sinacore DR, Siener C, Klein S. Effect of weight loss and exercise on frailty in obese older adults. Arch Intern Med 2006; 166(8): 860-6.
[http://dx.doi.org/10.1001/archinte.166.8.860] [PMID: 16636211]

[41] Miller SL, Wolfe RR. The danger of weight loss in the elderly. J Nutr Health Aging 2008; 12(7): 487-91.
[http://dx.doi.org/10.1007/BF02982710] [PMID: 18615231]

[42] Shapses SA, Riedt CS. Bone, body weight, and weight reduction: what are the concerns? J Nutr 2006; 136(6): 1453-6.
[PMID: 16702302]

[43] Shorr RI, Ray WA, Daugherty JR, Griffin MR. Individual sulfonylureas and serious hypoglycemia in older people. J Am Geriatr Soc 1996; 44(7): 751-5.
[http://dx.doi.org/10.1111/j.1532-5415.1996.tb03729.x] [PMID: 8675920]

[44] Hilmer SN, McLachlan AJ, Le Couteur DG. Clinical pharmacology in the geriatric patient. Fundam Clin Pharmacol 2007; 21(3): 217-30.
[http://dx.doi.org/10.1111/j.1472-8206.2007.00473.x] [PMID: 17521291]

[45] Stang M, Wysowski DK, Butler-Jones D. Incidence of lactic acidosis in metformin users. Diabetes Care 1999; 22(6): 925-7.
[http://dx.doi.org/10.2337/diacare.22.6.925] [PMID: 10372243]

[46] Lipska KJ, Bailey CJ, Inzucchi SE. Use of metformin in the setting of mild-to-moderate renal insufficiency. Diabetes Care 2011; 34(6): 1431-7.
[http://dx.doi.org/10.2337/dc10-2361] [PMID: 21617112]

[47] Graham GG, Punt J, Arora M, *et al.* Clinical pharmacokinetics of metformin. Clin Pharmacokinet 2011; 50(2): 81-98.
[http://dx.doi.org/10.2165/11534750-000000000-00000] [PMID: 21241070]

[48] Lee P, Chang A, Blaum C, Vlajnic A, Gao L, Halter J. Comparison of safety and efficacy of insulin glargine and neutral protamine hagedorn insulin in older adults with type 2 diabetes mellitus: results from a pooled analysis. J Am Geriatr Soc 2012; 60(1): 51-9.
[http://dx.doi.org/10.1111/j.1532-5415.2011.03773.x] [PMID: 22239291]

[49] Bolen S, Feldman L, Vassy J, *et al.* Systematic review: comparative effectiveness and safety of oral medications for type 2 diabetes mellitus. Ann Intern Med 2007; 147(6): 386-99.
[http://dx.doi.org/10.7326/0003-4819-147-6-200709180-00178] [PMID: 17638715]

[50] American Geriatrics Society updated Beers Criteria for potentially inappropriate medication use in

older adults. J Am Geriatr Soc 2012; 60(4): 616-31.
[http://dx.doi.org/10.1111/j.1532-5415.2012.03923.x] [PMID: 22376048]

[51] Berria R, Glass L, Mahankali A, *et al.* Reduction in hematocrit and hemoglobin following pioglitazone treatment is not hemodilutional in Type II diabetes mellitus. Clin Pharmacol Ther 2007; 82(3): 275-81.
[http://dx.doi.org/10.1038/sj.clpt.6100146] [PMID: 17361126]

[52] Graham DJ, Ouellet-Hellstrom R, MaCurdy TE, *et al.* Risk of acute myocardial infarction, stroke, heart failure, and death in elderly Medicare patients treated with rosiglitazone or pioglitazone. JAMA 2010; 304(4): 411-8.
[http://dx.doi.org/10.1001/jama.2010.920] [PMID: 20584880]

[53] Germino FW. Noninsulin treatment of type 2 diabetes mellitus in geriatric patients: a review. Clin Ther 2011; 33(12): 1868-82.
[http://dx.doi.org/10.1016/j.clinthera.2011.10.020] [PMID: 22136979]

[54] Schwarz SL, Gerich JE, Marcellari A, Jean-Louis L, Purkayastha D, Baron MA. Nateglinide, alone or in combination with metformin, is effective and well tolerated in treatment-naïve elderly patients with type 2 diabetes. Diabetes Obes Metab 2008; 10(8): 652-60.
[http://dx.doi.org/10.1111/j.1463-1326.2007.00792.x] [PMID: 17941876]

[55] Stein SA, Lamos EM, Davis SN. A review of the efficacy and safety of oral antidiabetic drugs. Expert Opin Drug Saf 2013; 12(2): 153-75.
[http://dx.doi.org/10.1517/14740338.2013.752813] [PMID: 23241069]

[56] Josse RG, Chiasson JL, Ryan EA, *et al.* Acarbose in the treatment of elderly patients with type 2 diabetes. Diabetes Res Clin Pract 2003; 59(1): 37-42.
[http://dx.doi.org/10.1016/S0168-8227(02)00176-6] [PMID: 12482640]

[57] Mooradian AD, Albert SG, Wittry S, Chehade J, Kim J, Bellrichard B. Dose-response profile of acarbose in older subjects with type 2 diabetes. Am J Med Sci 2000; 319(5): 334-7.
[http://dx.doi.org/10.1097/00000441-200005000-00011] [PMID: 10830558]

[58] Barnett AH, Huisman H, Jones R, von Eynatten M, Patel S, Woerle HJ. Linagliptin for patients aged 70 years or older with type 2 diabetes inadequately controlled with common antidiabetes treatments: a randomised, double-blind, placebo-controlled trial. Lancet 2013; 382(9902): 1413-23.
[http://dx.doi.org/10.1016/S0140-6736(13)61500-7] [PMID: 23948125]

[59] Karyekar CS, Ravichandran S, Allen E, Fleming D, Frederich R. Tolerability and efficacy of glycemic control with saxagliptin in older patients (aged ≥ 65 years) with inadequately controlled type 2 diabetes mellitus. Clin Interv Aging 2013; 8: 419-30.
[http://dx.doi.org/10.2147/CIA.S41246] [PMID: 23626461]

[60] Strain WD, Lukashevich V, Kothny W, Hoellinger MJ, Paldánius PM. Individualised treatment targets for elderly patients with type 2 diabetes using vildagliptin add-on or lone therapy (INTERVAL): a 24 week, randomised, double-blind, placebo-controlled study. Lancet 2013; 382(9890): 409-16.
[http://dx.doi.org/10.1016/S0140-6736(13)60995-2] [PMID: 23706759]

[61] Schweizer A, Dejager S. Experience with vildagliptin in patients ≥75 years with type 2 diabetes and moderate or severe renal impairment. Diabetes Ther 2013; 4(2): 257-67.
[http://dx.doi.org/10.1007/s13300-013-0027-x] [PMID: 23821355]

[62] Rosenstock J, Wilson C, Fleck P. Alogliptin *versus* glipizide monotherapy in elderly type 2 diabetes mellitus patients with mild hyperglycaemia: a prospective, double-blind, randomized, 1-year study. Diabetes Obes Metab 2013; 15(10): 906-14.
[http://dx.doi.org/10.1111/dom.12102] [PMID: 23531118]

[63] Round EM, Engel SS, Golm GT, Davies MJ, Kaufman KD, Goldstein BJ. Safety of sitagliptin in elderly patients with type 2 diabetes: a pooled analysis of 25 clinical studies. Drugs Aging 2014; 31(3): 203-14.
[http://dx.doi.org/10.1007/s40266-014-0155-7] [PMID: 24510656]

[64] Pawaskar M, Li Q, Reynolds MW. Metabolic outcomes of elderly patient populations initiating exenatide BID *versus* insulin glargine in an ambulatory care setting. Curr Med Res Opin 2012; 28(6): 991-7.
[http://dx.doi.org/10.1185/03007995.2012.686901] [PMID: 22519390]

[65] Thearle M, Brillantes AM. Unique characteristics of the geriatric diabetic population and the role for therapeutic strategies that enhance glucagon-like peptide-1 activity. Curr Opin Clin Nutr Metab Care 2005; 8(1): 9-16.
[http://dx.doi.org/10.1097/00075197-200501000-00003] [PMID: 15585995]

[66] Bode B, Stenlöf K, Sullivan D, Fung A, Usiskin K. Efficacy and safety of canagliflozin treatment in older subjects with type 2 diabetes mellitus: a randomized trial. Hosp Pract (1995) 2013; 41(2): 72-84.
[http://dx.doi.org/10.3810/hp.2013.04.1020] [PMID: 23680739]

[67] Yale JF, Bakris G, Cariou B, *et al.* Efficacy and safety of canagliflozin over 52 weeks in patients with type 2 diabetes mellitus and chronic kidney disease. Diabetes Obes Metab 2014; 16(10): 1016-27.
[http://dx.doi.org/10.1111/dom.12348] [PMID: 24965700]

[68] Singh-Franco D, Perez A, Harrington C. The effect of pramlintide acetate on glycemic control and weight in patients with type 2 diabetes mellitus and in obese patients without diabetes: a systematic review and meta-analysis. Diabetes Obes Metab 2011; 13(2): 169-80.
[http://dx.doi.org/10.1111/j.1463-1326.2010.01337.x] [PMID: 21199269]

[69] Herman WH, Ilag LL, Johnson SL, *et al.* A clinical trial of continuous subcutaneous insulin infusion *versus* multiple daily injections in older adults with type 2 diabetes. Diabetes Care 2005; 28(7): 1568-73.
[http://dx.doi.org/10.2337/diacare.28.7.1568] [PMID: 15983302]

[70] Bouillon K, Kivimäki M, Hamer M, *et al.* Diabetes risk factors, diabetes risk algorithms, and the prediction of future frailty: the Whitehall II prospective cohort study. J Am Med Dir Assoc 2013; 14(11): 851.e1-6.
[http://dx.doi.org/10.1016/j.jamda.2013.08.016] [PMID: 24103860]

[71] Espinoza SE, Jung I, Hazuda H. Frailty transitions in the San Antonio Longitudinal Study of Aging. J Am Geriatr Soc 2012; 60(4): 652-60.
[http://dx.doi.org/10.1111/j.1532-5415.2011.03882.x] [PMID: 22316162]

[72] Nouwen A, Winkley K, Twisk J, *et al.* Type 2 diabetes mellitus as a risk factor for the onset of depression: a systematic review and meta-analysis. Diabetologia 2010; 53(12): 2480-6.
[http://dx.doi.org/10.1007/s00125-010-1874-x] [PMID: 20711716]

[73] Lin EH, Katon W, Von Korff M, *et al.* Relationship of depression and diabetes self-care, medication adherence, and preventive care. Diabetes Care 2004; 27(9): 2154-60. [http://dx.doi.org/10.2337/diacare.27.9.2154] [PMID: 15333477]

[74] Black SA, Markides KS, Ray LA. Depression predicts increased incidence of adverse health outcomes in older Mexican Americans with type 2 diabetes. Diabetes Care 2003; 26(10): 2822-8. [http://dx.doi.org/10.2337/diacare.26.10.2822] [PMID: 14514586]

[75] Yesavage JA. Geriatric Depression Scale. Psychopharmacol Bull 1988; 24(4): 709-11. [PMID: 3249773]

[76] Rubin RR, Peyrot M. Psychosocial problems and interventions in diabetes. A review of the literature. Diabetes Care 1992; 15(11): 1640-57. [http://dx.doi.org/10.2337/diacare.15.11.1640] [PMID: 1468297]

[77] Cukierman T, Gerstein HC, Williamson JD. Cognitive decline and dementia in diabetes--systematic overview of prospective observational studies. Diabetologia 2005; 48(12): 2460-9. [http://dx.doi.org/10.1007/s00125-005-0023-4] [PMID: 16283246]

[78] Lu FP, Lin KP, Kuo HK. Diabetes and the risk of multi-system aging phenotypes: a systematic review and meta-analysis. PLoS One 2009; 4(1): e4144. [http://dx.doi.org/10.1371/journal.pone.0004144] [PMID: 19127292]

[79] Reaven GM, Thompson LW, Nahum D, Haskins E. Relationship between hyperglycemia and cognitive function in older NIDDM patients. Diabetes Care 1990; 13(1): 16-21. [http://dx.doi.org/10.2337/diacare.13.1.16] [PMID: 2298111]

[80] Araki A, Ito H. Asymptomatic cerebral infarction on brain MR images and cognitive function in elderly diabetic patients. Geriatr Gerontol Int 2002; 2: 206-14. [http://dx.doi.org/10.1046/j.1444-1586.2002.00047.x]

[81] Araki A, Ito H. Glucose metabolism, advanced glycation endproducts, and cognition. Geriatr Gerontol Int 2004; 4: S108-. [http://dx.doi.org/10.1111/j.1447-0594.2004.00169.x]

[82] Langan SJ, Deary IJ, Hepburn DA, Frier BM. Cumulative cognitive impairment following recurrent severe hypoglycaemia in adult patients with insulin-treated diabetes mellitus. Diabetologia 1991; 34(5): 337-44. [http://dx.doi.org/10.1007/BF00405006] [PMID: 1864488]

[83] Kalmijn S, Feskens EJ, Launer LJ, Stijnen T, Kromhout D. Glucose intolerance, hyperinsulinaemia and cognitive function in a general population of elderly men. Diabetologia 1995; 38(9): 1096-102. [http://dx.doi.org/10.1007/BF00402181] [PMID: 8591825]

[84] Sinclair AJ, Girling AJ, Bayer AJ. Cognitive dysfunction in older subjects with diabetes mellitus: impact on diabetes self-management and use of care services. All Wales Research into Elderly (AWARE) Study. Diabetes Res Clin Pract 2000; 50(3): 203-12. [http://dx.doi.org/10.1016/S0168-8227(00)00195-9] [PMID: 11106835]

[85] Gradman TJ, Laws A, Thompson LW, Reaven GM. Verbal learning and/or memory improves with glycemic control in older subjects with non-insulin-dependent diabetes mellitus. J Am Geriatr Soc 1993; 41(12): 1305-12.

[http://dx.doi.org/10.1111/j.1532-5415.1993.tb06480.x] [PMID: 8227912]

[86] Lifford KL, Curhan GC, Hu FB, Barbieri RL, Grodstein F. Type 2 diabetes mellitus and risk of developing urinary incontinence. J Am Geriatr Soc 2005; 53(11): 1851-7.
[http://dx.doi.org/10.1111/j.1532-5415.2005.53565.x] [PMID: 16274364]

[87] Jackson SL, Scholes D, Boyko EJ, Abraham L, Fihn SD. Urinary incontinence and diabetes in postmenopausal women. Diabetes Care 2005; 28(7): 1730-8.
[http://dx.doi.org/10.2337/diacare.28.7.1730] [PMID: 15983327]

[88] Brown JS, Vittinghoff E, Lin F, Nyberg LM, Kusek JW, Kanaya AM. Prevalence and risk factors for urinary incontinence in women with type 2 diabetes and impaired fasting glucose: findings from the National Health and Nutrition Examination Survey (NHANES) 2001-2002. Diabetes Care 2006; 29(6): 1307-12.
[http://dx.doi.org/10.2337/dc05-2463] [PMID: 16732013]

[89] Kim H, Yoshida H, Suzuki T. The effects of multidimensional exercise treatment on community-dwelling elderly Japanese women with stress, urge, and mixed urinary incontinence: a randomized controlled trial. Int J Nurs Stud 2011; 48(10): 1165-72.
[http://dx.doi.org/10.1016/j.ijnurstu.2011.02.016] [PMID: 21459381]

[90] van Houten P, Achterberg W, Ribbe M. Urinary incontinence in disabled elderly women: a randomized clinical trial on the effect of training mobility and toileting skills to achieve independent toileting. Gerontology 2007; 53(4): 205-10.
[http://dx.doi.org/10.1159/000100544] [PMID: 17347567]

[91] Gregg EW, Beckles GL, Williamson DF, *et al.* Diabetes and physical disability among older U.S. adults. Diabetes Care 2000; 23(9): 1272-7.
[http://dx.doi.org/10.2337/diacare.23.9.1272] [PMID: 10977018]

[92] Volpato S, Blaum C, Resnick H, Ferrucci L, Fried LP, Guralnik JM. Comorbidities and impairments explaining the association between diabetes and lower extremity disability: The Women's Health and Aging Study. Diabetes Care 2002; 25(4): 678-83.
[http://dx.doi.org/10.2337/diacare.25.4.678] [PMID: 11919124]

[93] Chipkin SR, Klugh SA, Chasan-Taber L. Exercise and diabetes. Cardiol Clin 2001; 19(3): 489-505.
[http://dx.doi.org/10.1016/S0733-8651(05)70231-9] [PMID: 11570119]

[94] Schwartz AV, Sellmeyer DE, Strotmeyer ES, *et al.* Diabetes and bone loss at the hip in older black and white adults. J Bone Miner Res 2005; 20(4): 596-603.
[http://dx.doi.org/10.1359/JBMR.041219] [PMID: 15765178]

[95] Volpato S, Leveille SG, Blaum C, Fried LP, Guralnik JM. Risk factors for falls in older disabled women with diabetes: the women's health and aging study. J Gerontol A Biol Sci Med Sci 2005; 60(12): 1539-45.
[http://dx.doi.org/10.1093/gerona/60.12.1539] [PMID: 16424285]

[96] Arvanitakis Z, Wilson RS, Schneider JA, Bienias JL, Evans DA, Bennett DA. Diabetes mellitus and progression of rigidity and gait disturbance in older persons. Neurology 2004; 63(6): 996-1001.
[http://dx.doi.org/10.1212/01.WNL.0000138432.16676.4B] [PMID: 15452289]

[97] Menz HB, Lord SR, St George R, Fitzpatrick RC. Walking stability and sensorimotor function in older

people with diabetic peripheral neuropathy. Arch Phys Med Rehabil 2004; 85(2): 245-52. [http://dx.doi.org/10.1016/j.apmr.2003.06.015] [PMID: 14966709]

[98] Costello E, Edelstein JE. Update on falls prevention for community-dwelling older adults: review of single and multifactorial intervention programs. J Rehabil Res Dev 2008; 45(8): 1135-52. [http://dx.doi.org/10.1682/JRRD.2007.10.0169] [PMID: 19235116]

[99] Matyka K, Evans M, Lomas J, Cranston I, Macdonald I, Amiel SA. Altered hierarchy of protective responses against severe hypoglycemia in normal aging in healthy men. Diabetes Care 1997; 20(2): 135-41. [http://dx.doi.org/10.2337/diacare.20.2.135] [PMID: 9118760]

[100] Chelliah A, Burge MR. Hypoglycaemia in elderly patients with diabetes mellitus: causes and strategies for prevention. Drugs Aging 2004; 21(8): 511-30. [http://dx.doi.org/10.2165/00002512-200421080-00003] [PMID: 15182216]

[101] Yun JS, Ko SH, Ko SH, *et al.* Presence of macroalbuminuria predicts severe hypoglycemia in patients with type 2 diabetes: a 10-year follow-up study. Diabetes Care 2013; 36(5): 1283-9. [http://dx.doi.org/10.2337/dc12-1408] [PMID: 23248198]

[102] Greco D, Pisciotta M, Gambina F, Maggio F. Severe hypoglycaemia leading to hospital admission in type 2 diabetic patients aged 80 years or older. Exp Clin Endocrinol Diabetes 2010; 118(4): 215-9. [http://dx.doi.org/10.1055/s-0029-1241823] [PMID: 20072965]

[103] Lipska KJ, Warton EM, Huang ES, *et al.* HbA1c and risk of severe hypoglycemia in type 2 diabetes: the Diabetes and Aging Study. Diabetes Care 2013; 36(11): 3535-42. [http://dx.doi.org/10.2337/dc13-0610] [PMID: 23900589]

Recent Advances in Geriatric Medicine, 2016, *Vol. 1*, 73-91

CHAPTER 5

Halting the Decline in Cognition: New Insights into Alzheimer's Disease

Kareeann Sok Fun Khow[1,*], Tuck Yean Yong[2]

[1] *Aged and Extended Care Services, The Queen Elizabeth Hospital and Department of Medicine, University of Adelaide, Adelaide, South Australia, Australia*

[2] *Internal Medicine, Flinders Private Hospital, Adelaide, South Australia, Australia*

Abstract: Alzheimer's disease is a major public health concern globally and has been identified as a research priority. Although this disease has been recognized for more than a century, there is an urgent need to improve our understanding of its pathogenesis in order to advance development of disease-modifying treatments. Clinical diagnosis of Alzheimer's disease remains the main method of identifying the disease but neuroimaging and biomarkers are emerging as adjunct tests in selective cases. Only a few pharmacological treatments are available for Alzheimer's disease and modest benefits are only observed in the mild-to-moderate disease. Without effective treatment, non-pharmacological approaches and prevention remain important. Non-pharmacological approaches such as exercise, cognitive stimulation therapy and computerized mind games are potentially beneficial in slowing the progression of Alzheimer's disease. Behavioural and psychological symptoms in Alzheimer's disease are still challenging to manage and require a combination of non-pharmacological and pharmacological approaches. Several novel therapies are currently under investigation and clinical trials of these agents will reveal if they are beneficial in the treatment of Alzheimer's disease.

Keywords: Alzheimer's disease, Anticholinesterase inhibitors, Behavioural symptoms, Carers, Cognitive impairment, Dementia, Diagnosis, Lifestyle modifications, Memantine, Psychological symptoms, Treatment.

* **Correspondence author Kareeann Sok Fun Khow:** Aged and Extended Care Services, The Queen Elizabeth Hospital, Woodville Road, Woodville South, South Australia 5011, Australia; Tel: +61 8 8222 6000; Fax: +61 8 8222 8593; E-mail: kareeann.khow@adelaide.edu.au.

Tuck Yean Yong (Ed)

INTRODUCTION

Alzheimer's disease is the most frequent cause of dementia in many countries. It was first named by Alois Alzheimer more than a century ago after examining a 51 year-old woman who was disoriented in time and place. He observed that "her ability to retain information is impaired to the profoundest degree" [1]. Interestingly in 2013, this patient's disease was finally understood when her DNA was found to have a rare mutation in the presenilin 1 gene that causes early onset Alzheimer's disease [2].

Alzheimer's disease has a significant impact on those with the condition as well as family and caregivers. Progression of the disease leads to loss of functional independence, the need for residential care and medical complications resulting in deaths.

EPIDEMIOLOGY

The Delphi study estimated that there were about 24 million people worldwide with dementia in 2001 and the majority are thought to have Alzheimer's disease [3]. It is predicted that the figure will rise to 42.3 million in 2020 and 81.1 million by 2040.

In 2010, 35.6 million people were estimated to have lived with dementia worldwide, with numbers predicted to increase two-fold every 20 years, to 65.7 million in 2030 and 115.4 million in 2050 [4]. In 2010, 58% of all people with dementia lived in countries with low or middle incomes, with this proportion anticipated to rise to 63% in 2030 and 71% in 2050.

RISK FACTORS

A consensus report from a panel of experts summarized some of the most consistently identified risk factors in Alzheimer's disease [5]. They found that smoking, depression, diabetes mellitus, metabolic syndrome and the apolipoprotein e4 (APOE e4) gene mutation were associated with increased risk of cognitive decline. The most prevalent genetic risk factor for late onset disease is the apolipoprotein ε4 allele, a gene for lipid transport in the brain. Over 65% of people with Alzheimer's disease are carriers of ε4 but only about 15% of the population possess it [6].

A family history of dementia is one of the most consistently reported risk factors for Alzheimer's disease [7]. Among patients with late-onset disease, first-degree relatives have about a two-fold increase in their lifetime risk of the disease [7]. In addition, the disease is more concordant in monozygotic twins than dizygotic twins [8]. Apart from genetic factors, many treatable medical conditions are also associated with an increased risk of Alzheimer's disease, including stroke, hypertension and hypercholesterolaemia [9 - 11].

PATHOGENESIS

There are three main hypotheses on the pathogenesis and aetiology of Alzheimer's disease: the amyloid plaques, neurofibrillary tangles and changes in neurotransmitter levels such as acetylcholine.

The amyloid hypothesis proposes that the pathological formation of amyloid plaques are directly toxic to cells and disrupt neurotransmission. These extracellular plaques are mainly made up of insoluble fibrils of amyloid beta (Aβ) peptide, which is formed when β-secretase and γ-secretase enzymes cleave amyloid precursor protein (APP). The ε4 allele is thought to promote deposition of Aβ [6]. However Aβ deposition does not correlate strongly with brain atrophy; nor is it detected consistently in people with early Alzheimer's-like neurodegeneration [12].

"Hyperphosphorylated" tau has been hypothesized as the cause of neurofibrillary tangles [13]. Tau, an insoluble protein, stabilises microtubules which in turn maintain the axons connecting neurons to one another. Hyperphosphorylated tau is thought to weaken axons because it does not bind to microtubules and it also forms protein filaments, which lead to neurofibrillary tangles. Neurofibrillary tangles correlate better with cognitive status and neuronal loss than the presence of amyloid plaques [14].

The third hypothesis focuses on the neurotransmitter acetylcholine. In people with Alzheimer's disease, less acetylcholine is present in their brains compared to those without dementia [15]. It is postulated that degeneration of the basal nucleus, the area of the brain that stimulates acetylcholine production and release, is responsible for this reduction. Another neurotransmitter in cortical areas involved in memory and learning is glutamate. In Alzheimer's disease, excess glutamate has been suggested to cause chronic activation of N-methyl-D-aspartate (NMDA) receptors, resulting in intracellular calcium overload and neuronal death from excitotoxicity [16].

DIAGNOSIS

Definite diagnosis of Alzheimer's disease can currently be made only at post-mortem. However, earlier diagnosis may be possible with new diagnostic investigations and criteria. Clinically it is only possible to make a probable diagnosis of the disease. This can be achieved by taking a thorough history of the symptoms and temporal patterns from the patient and other sources such as partner, carer or family members. Assessment is focused on determining the presence and severity of cognitive impairment and the effects on social, occupational and other instrumental functions. A neuropsychological assessment may also be included.

Typically the initial symptom of Alzheimer's disease involves an inability to retain recently learned information but memory of remote events is relatively spared until later. When the disease progresses, other cognitive areas such as language, abstract reasoning, executive function or decision making are impaired to varying degrees and this can lead to difficulty at work, social engagement or household activities. Deterioration in memory is often associated with changes in mood [17].

The Mini-Mental State Examination (MMSE) is one of the most commonly used tests for cognition, which has good sensitivity and specificity for dementia, but poor ability to recognize mild cognitive impairment [18, 19]. Using the MMSE, one study found that 25% of patients admitted to subacute care had dementia based on this test [20]. Among these, 70% were newly diagnosed after admission to subacute care.

An operationalised clinical approach with criteria such as the NINCDS-ADRDA (National Institute of Neurological and Communicative Disorders and Stroke and the Alzheimer's Disease and Related Disorders Association) has relatively good sensitivity (65%) and specificity (75%) for differentiating patients with probable Alzheimer's disease and those without dementia [21]. However its ability to differentiate between Alzheimer's disease and other forms of dementia is less precise (23-88%) [21].

BEHAVIOURAL AND PSYCHOLOGICAL SYMPTOMS

Behavioural and psychological symptoms of dementia (BPSD) include noncognitive symptoms and behaviours that commonly occur in patients with dementia [22]. Clinically significant BPSD are found in about 30% of community-dwelling people with dementia [23]. However this rises to almost 80% in people with dementia living in residential facilities [24]. BPSD symptoms tend to fluctuate. Symptom clusters include mood disorders (depression, anxiety and apathy/indifference), psychotic cluster (delusions and hallucinations), aberrant motor behaviours (pacing, wandering and other purposeless behaviours) and inappropriate behaviours (agitation, disinhibition and euphoria) [25]. The estimated proportion of patients with dementia affected by BPSD is shown in Table **1** [26 - 32]. BPSD are often associated with increased morbidity, increased cost of caring for the patient and decrease in quality of life for both patients and caregiver(s).

Table 1. Estimated proportion of patients with dementia affected by BPSD.

Symptom	Proportion of Patients with Dementia	References
Anxiety	24-65%	[26]
Apathy	48-92%	[26]
Delusions and hallucinations	9.2-36.0%	[27]
Depression	33-50%	[29, 30]
Disinhibition	36%	[26]
Euphoria	3.5-8.0%	[26, 33]
Irritability/mood lability/agitation	35-54%	[26]
Sleep disturbances	25%	[32]
Stereotyped behaviours (*e.g.*, pacing, wandering)	12-84%	[26]

NEUROIMAGING

According to evidence-based recommendations, CT or MRI are indicated if intracranial lesions or diseases that might cause or contribute to dementia syndromes (such as tumour, subdural haematomas, hydrocephalus or cerebrovascular disease) are clinically suspected [21].

Semi-quantitative structural MRI has been used to identify changes in medial temporal lobe atrophy between patients with Alzheimer's disease and age-matched control, with moderately high sensitivity and specificity of greater than 85% [21]. Furthermore, medial temporal atrophy has been proposed as a feature that can identify patients with mild cognitive impairment who will eventually progress to Alzheimer's disease. However, differences in medial temporal atrophy do not distinguish between Alzheimer's disease and non-Alzheimer's dementias.

Positron emission tomography (PET) with fluorodeoxyglucose has been found to have good accuracy in differentiating patients with probable Alzheimer's disease from both normal control people and those with non-Alzheimer's disease dementias [34]. A decrease of glucose metabolism in the temporal parietal regions and in the posterior cingulated cortex are findings commonly described in Alzheimer's disease. A meta-analysis has reported sensitivity and specificity of 86% for diagnosis of Alzheimer's disease with PET imaging but there were wide variations between studies [34]. Lower diagnostic values were found when distinguishing between Alzheimer's disease and non-Alzheimer's dementia [34]. A Cochrane systematic review analysed 14 studies evaluating the diagnostic accuracy of PET in determining the progression of mild cognitive impairment to Alzheimer's disease [35]. This review found that there was considerable variability of specificity values of PET and defined thresholds for test positivity was lacking and indicated that currently available evidence did not support the routine use of this imaging in people with mild cognitive impairment.

The use of amyloid PET in Alzheimer's disease was first reported in 2004 [36]. A systematic review has found that amyloid PET had a sensitivity and specificity of 85% in differentiating Alzheimer's disease from absence of the disorder [37]. However the specificity of this imaging approach was only 46-88% for identifying those with mild cognitive impairment who will progress to Alzheimer's disease [38].

OTHER INVESTIGATIONS

Studies have found that analysis of Aβ peptide, tau and other compounds in the cerebrospinal fluid (CSF) can be combined to give >90% sensitivity and >80% specificity in predicting progression of mild cognitive impairment to Alzheimer's disease or distinguishing Alzheimer's from other forms of dementias [39, 40]. However, a Cochrane systematic review found that abnormally low CSF Aβ levels has little diagnostic value in predicting the progression of mild cognitive impairment to Alzheimer's disease [41]. Blood concentrations of Aβ peptide and tau are unreliable diagnostic tests. In terms of a peripheral blood test, a study has found 10 lipid metabolites to have >90% sensitivity and specificity in predicting who would develop mild cognitive impairment or Alzheimer's disease [42]. However, this test requires further validation.

NATURAL HISTORY

The onset of Alzheimer's disease is usually insidious and manifestations gradually evolve over a period of years from mild memory impairment to severe cognitive loss. Mild cognitive impairment often precedes the earliest manifestation of Alzheimer's disease [43]. The course of this disease is generally progressive and results in mental and functional disability and eventually death. Plateaus sometimes occur with stabilization of cognitive impairment for one to two years but progression usually follows thereafter.

MANAGEMENT – NON-PHARMACOLOGICAL THERAPY

For people living in nursing homes, dementia is an important predictor of walking ability, functional status and mortality [44]. However, physical exercise can be a major therapy in Alzheimer's disease. In one study, resistance exercises improved the Alzheimer Disease Assessment Scale-Cognition and slowed deterioration in executive function [45]. Exercise can also reduce difficult behavioural expression in nursing home residents with dementia [46].

Computerized mind games have a small effect on improving cognition in

Alzheimer's disease [47]. There is also some evidence that reminiscence therapy can improve cognition [48, 49]. Cognitive stimulation therapy is also thought to be effective not only for improving cognition but also quality of life [50, 51]. To effectively manage people with Alzheimer's disease, patients and families should be involved as soon as the diagnosis is made.

MANAGEMENT – PHARMACOLOGICAL THERAPY

The main class of drugs for Alzheimer's disease has been the cholinesterase inhibitors, which inhibit the breakdown of acetylcholine. Donepezil, galantamine and rivastigmine are among the most commonly used cholinesterase inhibitors for mild-to-moderate disease (Table **2**). Evidence from clinical trials and clinical practice indicate improvement on cognition is moderate (1.5-2 points on the MMSE over 6-12 months) with additional short-term (3-6 months) improvement in global outcome and stabilisation of functional status over this period [52 - 55]. Modest improvements in mood especially apathy, and social interaction have been reported with cholinesterase inhibitors [53 - 55].

Table 2. Pharmacological treatments used in Alzheimer's disease.

	Drugs	**Evidence**
Cognition-modifying treatment		
Cholinesterase inhibitors	Donepezil, rivastigmine, galantamine	Significant benefits in cognition, function and global outcome, with MMSE gain of 1.5-2 points over 6-12 months in mild-to-moderate Alzheimer's disease.
NMDA	Memantine	Significant benefit in cognition, function, global outcome and neuropsychiatric symptoms over 6 months in moderate-to-severe Alzheimer's disease
Treatment for neuropsychiatric symptoms		
Atypical antipsychotics	Risperidone, quetiapine, olanzapine, aripiprazole	Moderate efficacy for treatment of aggression and psychosis over 6-12 weeks. Limited evidence for long-term benefits. Atypical antipsychotics associated with increased risk of stroke and death.
Antidepressants	Citalopram, sertraline	No convincing evidence for neuropyschiatric symptoms in Alzheimer's disease.

(Table 2) contd.....

	Drugs	Evidence
Anticonvulsants	Carbamazepine	Insufficient evidence to recommend routine use of carbamazepine in treatment of BPSD.

MANAGEMENT – BEHAVIOURAL AND PSYCHOLOGICAL SYMPTOMS

Effective treatment strategies for BPSD include various nonpharmacological and pharmacological approaches. Nonpharmacological treatments found to be effective in BPSD include psychoeducation of caregivers, behaviour therapy and multisensory therapy [56, 57]. Current evidence indicate short-term efficacy for atypical antipsychotics, especially risperidone, aripiprazole, and to a lesser extent, olanzapine, in the management of BPSD (Table **2**) [58, 59]. Evidence indicates that these antipsychotics generally should not be used for longer than 12 weeks but long-term therapy may be needed in some patients who have persistent symptoms even though data for longer duration of treatment is limited [58 - 61]. Antipsychotics should be prescribed within the recommended dose ranges to minimise the risk of serious adverse events such as cerebrovascular events and death [62]. Alternatives to antipsychotics in managing BPSD include anticonvulsants, antidepressants, cholinesterase inhibitors and memantine but these drugs may have better efficacy in treating nonaggressive behaviours such as apathy than in treating agitation, aggression and psychotic symptoms such as delusions and hallucinations [63 - 65].

PROPOSED TREATMENT

New treatments targeting Aβ peptide has not achieved as much benefit as initially envisaged. A trial of active immunisation with the first Aβ vaccine was ceased after 6% of participants unexpectedly developed meningoencephalitis and a later analysis did not reveal any clinical benefit [66, 67]. Phase 3 trials of two monoclonal antibodies against Aβ, solanezumab and bapineuzumab, also did not meet primary endpoints of improvement in cognitive function [68, 69].

Studies using γ-secretase inhibitors, semagacestat and avagacestat, have also shown unconvincing improvement in outcomes [70, 71]. Another agent, tramiprosate, has been trialled but no clinical benefit was shown [72]. Currently β-secretase inhibitors are under development [73]. Trials are also in progress for drugs that inhibit phosphorylation of tau and antibodies against tau [74].

CAREGIVERS

A timely diagnosis offers caregivers the opportunity to adapt to the caregiver role. Caregivers who are better able to adapt to the changes observed in people with Alzheimer's disease, feel more competent to care and experience less psychological problems. However, benefits of an early diagnosis has to be balanced with problems arising if people are left with a diagnosis but little support. There is moderately strong evidence that multicomponent caregiver interventions in the milder stages of dementia are effective in improving caregiver well-being and delay institutionalization. However, there is still a gap between the improved possibilities to diagnose people in the early stage and the scarce knowledge on intervention effects in this very early stage. Therefore there is a pressing need for more research on early caregiver interventions that enhance role adaptation, which includes long-term follow-up and cost-effectiveness evaluation.

Whenever possible, caregivers should be encouraged to come to all of the patients' appointments to ensure the safe arrival of patients and to facilitate accurate assessment of symptoms. In addition, this also provides an opportunity for the caregivers' own level of stress to be assessed. Early interventions may help caregivers in anticipating and accepting the future care role and transitions, with the increased possibility that caregivers can still involve the patient in the decision making process. As levels of stress and burden are still low in the early stage it provides excellent opportunities to equip caregivers with resources to meet anticipated future needs.

People who provide care for patients with Alzheimer's disease often report emotional stress, in part related to the need to give up vacations, change of life routines, or even work to care for the patient. Severity of psychiatric symptoms, behavioral disturbances, and patients' quality of life have been reported to correlate with caregivers' experience of burden [75]. Therefore, psychosocial and pharmacological interventions targeting these aspects of the disorder are beneficial in alleviating patient suffering but promoting caregiver well-being.

Caregivers should routinely be offered counselling and support. Resources for caregivers and patients should be made available through local Alzheimer's disease support groups.

STRATEGIES TO PREVENT ALZHEIMER'S DISEASE

Without effective pharmacological therapy against this disease, prevention remains important. This is best achieved by developing a "cognitive reserve" in early life through educational and occupational stimulation. Maintenance of this reserve depends on continuing cognitively stimulating activities and social engagement, as well as avoiding recognised risk factors such as lack of exercise, smoking, excessive alcohol, poor diet, hypertension, diabetes and obesity [76 - 78]. Based on available evidence, vitamin supplements are ineffective but several cohort studies have supported the protective effects of a Mediterranean diet to reduce the risk of Alzheimer's disease [79].

GAPS IN CURRENT EVIDENCE AND FUTURE RESEARCH

Despite recent advances, there is still a considerable gap in the understanding of the pathogenesis of Alzheimer's disease. Early identification and accurate diagnosis of Alzheimer's disease remains a problem in both clinical and research settings. Further study of brain imaging and biomarkers may facilitate the early identification of patients with Alzheimer's disease. One of the greatest needs in Alzheimer's disease research is to identify effective pharmacological intervention.

CONCLUSION

Alzhiemer's disease is the commonest cause of dementia but remains a perplexing problem for patients and health care professionals. Early identification and accurate diagnosis of Alzheimer's disease is still a recurring problem even in research settings. Despite advances in diagnostic neuroimaging, these new techniques are still too expensive and not accurate enough for routine clinical use. At best, current therapies for patients with Alzheimer's disease may provide temporary improvement and reduce the rate of cognitive decline. As new molecular targets are being identified, it is hoped that new interventions can be developed to modify the progression of this disease. In the absence of disease-modifying therapy, preventive strategies such as treatment of cardiovascular risk factors, are important.

CONFLICT OF INTEREST

The author confirms that author has no conflict of interest to declare for this publication.

ACKNOWLEDGEMENTS

Declared none.

KEY POINTS

- Clinically it is only possible to make a probable diagnosis of Alzheimer's disease.
- New neuroimaging techniques are promising tools for the evaluation of Alzheimer's disease but are currently not recommended for routine clinical use.
- Anticholinesterase inhibitors and memantine may slow the rate of cognitive decline in Alzheimer's disease but disease-modifying therapy is still lacking.
- Lifestyle modification and exercise are important adjunct therapy in the management of Alzheimer's disease.
- Management of behavioural and psychological symptoms in Alzheimer's disease should involve both non-pharmacological and pharmacological approaches.

REFERENCES

[1] Strassnig M, Ganguli M. About a peculiar disease of the cerebral cortex: Alzheimer's original case revisited. Psychiatry (Edgmont) 2005; 2(9): 30-3.
[PMID: 21120106]

[2] Müller U, Winter P, Graeber MB. A presenilin 1 mutation in the first case of Alzheimer's disease. Lancet Neurol 2013; 12(2): 129-30.
[http://dx.doi.org/10.1016/S1474-4422(12)70307-1] [PMID: 23246540]

[3] Ferri CP, Prince M, Brayne C, *et al.* Global prevalence of dementia: a Delphi consensus study. Lancet 2005; 366(9503): 2112-7.
[http://dx.doi.org/10.1016/S0140-6736(05)67889-0] [PMID: 16360788]

[4] Prince M, Bryce R, Albanese E, Wimo A, Ribeiro W, Ferri CP. The global prevalence of dementia: a systematic review and metaanalysis. Alzheimers Dement 2013; 9(1): 63-75.e2.

[http://dx.doi.org/10.1016/j.jalz.2012.11.007] [PMID: 23305823]

[5] Plassman BL, Williams JW Jr, Burke JR, Holsinger T, Benjamin S. Systematic review: factors associated with risk for and possible prevention of cognitive decline in later life. Ann Intern Med 2010; 153(3): 182-93.
[http://dx.doi.org/10.7326/0003-4819-153-3-201008030-00258] [PMID: 20547887]

[6] Huang Y. Abeta-independent roles of apolipoprotein E4 in the pathogenesis of Alzheimer's disease. Trends Mol Med 2010; 16(6): 287-94.
[http://dx.doi.org/10.1016/j.molmed.2010.04.004] [PMID: 20537952]

[7] Rogaeva E, Kawarai T, George-Hyslop PS. Genetic complexity of Alzheimer's disease: successes and challenges. J Alzheimers Dis 2006; 9(3) (Suppl.): 381-7.
[PMID: 16914876]

[8] Gatz M, Reynolds CA, Fratiglioni L, *et al.* Role of genes and environments for explaining Alzheimer disease. Arch Gen Psychiatry 2006; 63(2): 168-74.
[http://dx.doi.org/10.1001/archpsyc.63.2.168] [PMID: 16461860]

[9] Qiu C, Winblad B, Fratiglioni L. The age-dependent relation of blood pressure to cognitive function and dementia. Lancet Neurol 2005; 4(8): 487-99.
[http://dx.doi.org/10.1016/S1474-4422(05)70141-1] [PMID: 16033691]

[10] Savva GM, Stephan BC. Epidemiological studies of the effect of stroke on incident dementia: a systematic review. Stroke 2010; 41(1): e41-6.
[http://dx.doi.org/10.1161/STROKEAHA.109.559880] [PMID: 19910553]

[11] Kivipelto M, Solomon A. Cholesterol as a risk factor for Alzheimer's disease - epidemiological evidence. Acta Neurol Scand Suppl 2006; 185: 50-7.
[http://dx.doi.org/10.1111/j.1600-0404.2006.00685.x] [PMID: 16866911]

[12] Zetterberg H, Mattsson N. Understanding the cause of sporadic Alzheimer's disease. Expert Rev Neurother 2014; 14(6): 621-30.
[http://dx.doi.org/10.1586/14737175.2014.915740] [PMID: 24852227]

[13] Grundke-Iqbal I, Iqbal K, Tung YC, Quinlan M, Wisniewski HM, Binder LI. Abnormal phosphorylation of the microtubule-associated protein tau (tau) in Alzheimer cytoskeletal pathology. Proc Natl Acad Sci USA 1986; 83(13): 4913-7.
[http://dx.doi.org/10.1073/pnas.83.13.4913] [PMID: 3088567]

[14] Giannakopoulos P, Herrmann FR, Bussière T, *et al.* Tangle and neuron numbers, but not amyloid load, predict cognitive status in Alzheimer's disease. Neurology 2003; 60(9): 1495-500.
[http://dx.doi.org/10.1212/01.WNL.0000063311.58879.01] [PMID: 12743238]

[15] Harrison PJ. Pathogenesis of Alzheimer's disease--beyond the cholinergic hypothesis: discussion paper. J R Soc Med 1986; 79(6): 347-52.
[PMID: 2873250]

[16] Danysz W, Parsons CG. Alzheimer's disease, β-amyloid, glutamate, NMDA receptors and memantine--searching for the connections. Br J Pharmacol 2012; 167(2): 324-52.
[http://dx.doi.org/10.1111/j.1476-5381.2012.02057.x] [PMID: 22646481]

[17] Ownby RL, Crocco E, Acevedo A, John V, Loewenstein D. Depression and risk for Alzheimer

disease: systematic review, meta-analysis, and metaregression analysis. Arch Gen Psychiatry 2006; 63(5): 530-8.
[http://dx.doi.org/10.1001/archpsyc.63.5.530] [PMID: 16651510]

[18] Kaufer DI, Williams CS, Braaten AJ, Gill K, Zimmerman S, Sloane PD. Cognitive screening for dementia and mild cognitive impairment in assisted living: comparison of 3 tests. J Am Med Dir Assoc 2008; 9(8): 586-93.
[http://dx.doi.org/10.1016/j.jamda.2008.05.006] [PMID: 19083293]

[19] Cruz-Oliver DM, Morley JE. Early detection of cognitive impairment: do screening tests help? J Am Med Dir Assoc 2010; 11(1): 1-6.
[http://dx.doi.org/10.1016/j.jamda.2009.10.012] [PMID: 20129206]

[20] Ferretti M, Seematter-Bagnoud L, Martin E, Büla CJ. New diagnoses of dementia among older patients admitted to postacute care. J Am Med Dir Assoc 2010; 11(5): 371-6.
[http://dx.doi.org/10.1016/j.jamda.2009.10.002] [PMID: 20511105]

[21] Waldemar G, Dubois B, Emre M, *et al.* Recommendations for the diagnosis and management of Alzheimer's disease and other disorders associated with dementia: EFNS guideline. Eur J Neurol 2007; 14(1): e1-e26.
[http://dx.doi.org/10.1111/j.1468-1331.2006.01605.x] [PMID: 17222085]

[22] Lawlor B. Managing behavioural and psychological symptoms in dementia. Br J Psychiatry 2002; 181: 463-5.
[http://dx.doi.org/10.1192/bjp.181.6.463] [PMID: 12456513]

[23] Lyketsos CG, Steinberg M, Tschanz JT, Norton MC, Steffens DC, Breitner JC. Mental and behavioral disturbances in dementia: findings from the Cache County Study on Memory in Aging. Am J Psychiatry 2000; 157(5): 708-14.
[http://dx.doi.org/10.1176/appi.ajp.157.5.708] [PMID: 10784462]

[24] Margallo-Lana M, Swann A, O'Brien J, *et al.* Prevalence and pharmacological management of behavioural and psychological symptoms amongst dementia sufferers living in care environments. Int J Geriatr Psychiatry 2001; 16(1): 39-44.
[http://dx.doi.org/10.1002/1099-1166(200101)16:1<39::AID-GPS269>3.0.CO;2-F] [PMID: 11180484]

[25] Cummings JL, Back C. The cholinergic hypothesis of neuropsychiatric symptoms in Alzheimer's disease. Am J Geriatr Psychiatry 1998; 6(2) (Suppl. 1): S64-78.
[http://dx.doi.org/10.1097/00019442-199821001-00009] [PMID: 9581223]

[26] Mega MS, Masterman DM, O'Connor SM, Barclay TR, Cummings JL. The spectrum of behavioral responses to cholinesterase inhibitor therapy in Alzheimer disease. Arch Neurol 1999; 56(11): 1388-93.
[http://dx.doi.org/10.1001/archneur.56.11.1388] [PMID: 10555660]

[27] Bassiony MM, Steinberg MS, Warren A, Rosenblatt A, Baker AS, Lyketsos CG. Delusions and hallucinations in Alzheimer's disease: prevalence and clinical correlates. Int J Geriatr Psychiatry 2000; 15(2): 99-107.
[http://dx.doi.org/10.1002/(SICI)1099-1166(200002)15:2<99::AID-GPS82>3.0.CO;2-5] [PMID: 10679840]

[28] Ropacki SA, Jeste DV. Epidemiology of and risk factors for psychosis of Alzheimer's disease: a review of 55 studies published from 1990 to 2003. Am J Psychiatry 2005; 162(11): 2022-30. [http://dx.doi.org/10.1176/appi.ajp.162.11.2022] [PMID: 16263838]

[29] Lee HB, Lyketsos CG. Depression in Alzheimer's disease: heterogeneity and related issues. Biol Psychiatry 2003; 54(3): 353-62. [http://dx.doi.org/10.1016/S0006-3223(03)00543-2] [PMID: 12893110]

[30] Olin JT, Katz IR, Meyers BS, Schneider LS, Lebowitz BD. Provisional diagnostic criteria for depression of Alzheimer disease: rationale and background. Am J Geriatr Psychiatry 2002; 10(2): 129-41. [http://dx.doi.org/10.1097/00019442-200203000-00004] [PMID: 11925274]

[31] Burns A, Jacoby R, Levy R. Psychiatric phenomena in Alzheimer's disease. III: Disorders of mood. Br J Psychiatry 1990; 157: 81-86, 92-94. [http://dx.doi.org/10.1192/bjp.157.1.81] [PMID: 2397367]

[32] Rose KM, Lorenz R. Sleep disturbances in dementia. J Gerontol Nurs 2010; 36(5): 9-14. [http://dx.doi.org/10.3928/00989134-20100330-05] [PMID: 20438013]

[33] Burns A, Jacoby R, Levy R. Psychiatric phenomena in Alzheimer's disease. IV: Disorders of behaviour. Br J Psychiatry 1990; 157: 86-94. [http://dx.doi.org/10.1192/bjp.157.1.86] [PMID: 2397368]

[34] Patwardhan MB, McCrory DC, Matchar DB, Samsa GP, Rutschmann OT. Alzheimer disease: operating characteristics of PET--a meta-analysis. Radiology 2004; 231(1): 73-80. [http://dx.doi.org/10.1148/radiol.2311021620] [PMID: 15068942]

[35] Smailagic N, Vacante M, Hyde C, Martin S, Ukoumunne O, Sachpekidis C. ^{18}F-FDG PET for the early diagnosis of Alzheimer's disease dementia and other dementias in people with mild cognitive impairment (MCI). Cochrane Database Syst Rev 2015; 1: CD010632. [http://dx.doi.org/10.1148/radiol.2311021620] [PMID: 25629415]

[36] Klunk WE, Engler H, Nordberg A, *et al.* Imaging brain amyloid in Alzheimer's disease with Pittsburgh Compound-B. Ann Neurol 2004; 55(3): 306-19. [http://dx.doi.org/10.1002/ana.20009] [PMID: 14991808]

[37] Frisoni GB, Bocchetta M, Chételat G, *et al.* Imaging markers for Alzheimer disease: which *vs* how. Neurology 2013; 81(5): 487-500. [http://dx.doi.org/10.1212/WNL.0b013e31829d86e8] [PMID: 23897875]

[38] Zhang S, Smailagic N, Hyde C, *et al.* (11)C-PIB-PET for the early diagnosis of Alzheimer's disease dementia and other dementias in people with mild cognitive impairment (MCI). Cochrane Database Syst Rev 2014; 7: CD010386. [PMID: 25052054]

[39] Hansson O, Zetterberg H, Buchhave P, Londos E, Blennow K, Minthon L. Association between CSF biomarkers and incipient Alzheimer's disease in patients with mild cognitive impairment: a follow-up study. Lancet Neurol 2006; 5(3): 228-34. [http://dx.doi.org/10.1016/S1474-4422(06)70355-6] [PMID: 16488378]

[40] Welge V, Fiege O, Lewczuk P, *et al.* Combined CSF tau, p-tau181 and amyloid-beta 38/40/42 for

diagnosing Alzheimer's disease. J Neural Transm (Vienna) 2009; 116(2): 203-12. [http://dx.doi.org/10.1007/s00702-008-0177-6] [PMID: 19142572]

[41] Ritchie C, Smailagic N, Noel-Storr AH, *et al.* Plasma and cerebrospinal fluid amyloid beta for the diagnosis of Alzheimer's disease dementia and other dementias in people with mild cognitive impairment (MCI). Cochrane Database Syst Rev 2014; 6: CD008782. [PMID: 24913723]

[42] Mapstone M, Cheema AK, Fiandaca MS, *et al.* Plasma phospholipids identify antecedent memory impairment in older adults. Nat Med 2014; 20(4): 415-8. [http://dx.doi.org/10.1038/nm.3466] [PMID: 24608097]

[43] Petersen RC, Doody R, Kurz A, *et al.* Current concepts in mild cognitive impairment. Arch Neurol 2001; 58(12): 1985-92. [http://dx.doi.org/10.1001/archneur.58.12.1985] [PMID: 11735772]

[44] González-Colaço Harmand M, Meillon C, Rullier L, *et al.* Cognitive decline after entering a nursing home: a 22-year follow-up study of institutionalized and noninstitutionalized elderly people. J Am Med Dir Assoc 2014; 15(7): 504-8. [http://dx.doi.org/10.1016/j.jamda.2014.02.006] [PMID: 24679926]

[45] Fiatarone Singh MA, Gates N, Saigal N, *et al.* The Study of Mental and Resistance Training (SMART) study—resistance training and/or cognitive training in mild cognitive impairment: a randomized, double-blind, double-sham controlled trial. J Am Med Dir Assoc 2014; 15(12): 873-80. [http://dx.doi.org/10.1016/j.jamda.2014.09.010] [PMID: 25444575]

[46] Aman E, Thomas DR. Supervised exercise to reduce agitation in severely cognitively impaired persons. J Am Med Dir Assoc 2009; 10(4): 271-6. [http://dx.doi.org/10.1016/j.jamda.2008.12.053] [PMID: 19426944]

[47] Anderson K, Grossberg GT. Brain games to slow cognitive decline in Alzheimer's disease. J Am Med Dir Assoc 2014; 15(8): 536-7. [http://dx.doi.org/10.1016/j.jamda.2014.04.014] [PMID: 24913208]

[48] Van Bogaert P, Van Grinsven R, Tolson D, Wouters K, Engelborghs S, Van der Mussele S. Effects of SolCos model-based individual reminiscence on older adults with mild to moderate dementia due to Alzheimer disease: a pilot study. J Am Med Dir Assoc 2013; 14(7): 528-41.

[49] Wingbermuehle C, Bryer D, Berg-Weger M, *et al.* Baseball reminiscence league: a model for supporting persons with dementia. J Am Med Dir Assoc 2014; 15(2): 85-9. [http://dx.doi.org/10.1016/j.jamda.2013.11.006] [PMID: 24461238]

[50] Woods B, Aguirre E, Spector AE, Orrell M. Cognitive stimulation to improve cognitive functioning in people with dementia. Cochrane Database Syst Rev 2012; 2: CD005562. [PMID: 22336813]

[51] Aguirre E, Woods RT, Spector A, Orrell M. Cognitive stimulation for dementia: a systematic review of the evidence of effectiveness from randomised controlled trials. Ageing Res Rev 2013; 12(1): 253-62. [http://dx.doi.org/10.1016/j.arr.2012.07.001] [PMID: 22889599]

[52] Birks J, Harvey RJ. Donepezil for dementia due to Alzheimer's disease. Cochrane Database Syst Rev

2006; (1): CD001190.
[PMID: 16437430]

[53] Birks J. Cholinesterase inhibitors for Alzheimer's disease. Cochrane Database Syst Rev 2006; (1): CD005593.
[PMID: 16437532]

[54] Loy C, Schneider L. Galantamine for Alzheimer's disease and mild cognitive impairment. Cochrane Database Syst Rev 2006; (1): CD001747.
[PMID: 16437436]

[55] Birks J, Grimley Evans J, Iakovidou V, Tsolaki M, Holt FE. Rivastigmine for Alzheimer's disease. Cochrane Database Syst Rev 2009; (2): CD001191.
[PMID: 19370562]

[56] Verkaik R, van Weert JC, Francke AL. The effects of psychosocial methods on depressed, aggressive and apathetic behaviors of people with dementia: a systematic review. Int J Geriatr Psychiatry 2005; 20(4): 301-14.
[http://dx.doi.org/10.1002/gps.1279] [PMID: 15799081]

[57] Livingston G, Johnston K, Katona C, Paton J, Lyketsos CG. Systematic review of psychological approaches to the management of neuropsychiatric symptoms of dementia. Am J Psychiatry 2005; 162(11): 1996-2021.
[http://dx.doi.org/10.1176/appi.ajp.162.11.1996] [PMID: 16263837]

[58] Ballard C, Waite J. The effectiveness of atypical antipsychotics for the treatment of aggression and psychosis in Alzheimer's disease. Cochrane Database Syst Rev 2006; (1): CD003476.
[PMID: 16437455]

[59] Schneider LS, Dagerman K, Insel PS. Efficacy and adverse effects of atypical antipsychotics for dementia: meta-analysis of randomized, placebo-controlled trials. Am J Geriatr Psychiatry 2006; 14(3): 191-210.
[http://dx.doi.org/10.1097/01.JGP.0000200589.01396.6d] [PMID: 16505124]

[60] Schneider LS, Dagerman KS, Insel P. Risk of death with atypical antipsychotic drug treatment for dementia: meta-analysis of randomized placebo-controlled trials. JAMA 2005; 294(15): 1934-43.
[http://dx.doi.org/10.1001/jama.294.15.1934] [PMID: 16234500]

[61] Schneider LS, Tariot PN, Dagerman KS, *et al.* Effectiveness of atypical antipsychotic drugs in patients with Alzheimer's disease. N Engl J Med 2006; 355(15): 1525-38.
[http://dx.doi.org/10.1056/NEJMoa061240] [PMID: 17035647]

[62] Mittal V, Kurup L, Williamson D, Muralee S, Tampi RR. Risk of cerebrovascular adverse events and death in elderly patients with dementia when treated with antipsychotic medications: a literature review of evidence. Am J Alzheimers Dis Other Demen 2011; 26(1): 10-28.
[http://dx.doi.org/10.1177/1533317510390351] [PMID: 21282274]

[63] Konovalov S, Muralee S, Tampi RR. Anticonvulsants for the treatment of behavioral and psychological symptoms of dementia: a literature review. Int Psychogeriatr 2008; 20(2): 293-308.
[http://dx.doi.org/10.1017/S1041610207006540] [PMID: 18047764]

[64] Trinh NH, Hoblyn J, Mohanty S, Yaffe K. Efficacy of cholinesterase inhibitors in the treatment of

neuropsychiatric symptoms and functional impairment in Alzheimer disease: a meta-analysis. JAMA 2003; 289(2): 210-6.
[http://dx.doi.org/10.1001/jama.289.2.210] [PMID: 12517232]

[65] Maidment ID, Fox CG, Boustani M, Rodriguez J, Brown RC, Katona CL. Efficacy of memantine on behavioral and psychological symptoms related to dementia: a systematic meta-analysis. Ann Pharmacother 2008; 42(1): 32-8.
[http://dx.doi.org/10.1345/aph.1K372] [PMID: 18056833]

[66] Orgogozo JM, Gilman S, Dartigues JF, *et al.* Subacute meningoencephalitis in a subset of patients with AD after Abeta42 immunization. Neurology 2003; 61(1): 46-54.
[http://dx.doi.org/10.1212/01.WNL.0000073623.84147.A8] [PMID: 12847155]

[67] Holmes C, Boche D, Wilkinson D, *et al.* Long-term effects of Abeta42 immunisation in Alzheimer's disease: follow-up of a randomised, placebo-controlled phase I trial. Lancet 2008; 372(9634): 216-23.
[http://dx.doi.org/10.1016/S0140-6736(08)61075-2] [PMID: 18640458]

[68] Doody RS, Thomas RG, Farlow M, *et al.* Phase 3 trials of solanezumab for mild-to-moderate Alzheimer's disease. N Engl J Med 2014; 370(4): 311-21.
[http://dx.doi.org/10.1056/NEJMoa1312889] [PMID: 24450890]

[69] Salloway S, Sperling R, Fox NC, *et al.* Two phase 3 trials of bapineuzumab in mild-to-moderate Alzheimer's disease. N Engl J Med 2014; 370(4): 322-33.
[http://dx.doi.org/10.1056/NEJMoa1304839] [PMID: 24450891]

[70] Coric V, van Dyck CH, Salloway S, *et al.* Safety and tolerability of the γ-secretase inhibitor avagacestat in a phase 2 study of mild to moderate Alzheimer disease. Arch Neurol 2012; 69(11): 1430-40.
[http://dx.doi.org/10.1001/archneurol.2012.2194] [PMID: 22892585]

[71] Doody RS, Raman R, Farlow M, *et al.* A phase 3 trial of semagacestat for treatment of Alzheimer's disease. N Engl J Med 2013; 369(4): 341-50.
[http://dx.doi.org/10.1056/NEJMoa1210951] [PMID: 23883379]

[72] Aisen PS, Gauthier S, Ferris SH, *et al.* Tramiprosate in mild-to-moderate Alzheimer's disease - a randomized, double-blind, placebo-controlled, multi-centre study (the Alphase Study). Arch Med Sci 2011; 7(1): 102-11.
[http://dx.doi.org/10.5114/aoms.2011.20612] [PMID: 22291741]

[73] Nygaard HB. Current and emerging therapies for Alzheimer's disease. Clin Ther 2013; 35(10): 1480-9.
[http://dx.doi.org/10.1016/j.clinthera.2013.09.009] [PMID: 24139420]

[74] Giacobini E, Gold G. Alzheimer disease therapy--moving from amyloid-β to tau. Nat Rev Neurol 2013; 9(12): 677-86.
[http://dx.doi.org/10.1038/nrneurol.2013.223] [PMID: 24217510]

[75] Mohamed S, Rosenheck R, Lyketsos CG, Schneider LS. Caregiver burden in Alzheimer disease: cross-sectional and longitudinal patient correlates. Am J Geriatr Psychiatry 2010; 18(10): 917-27.
[http://dx.doi.org/10.1097/JGP.0b013e3181d5745d] [PMID: 20808108]

[76] Middleton LE, Yaffe K. Promising strategies for the prevention of dementia. Arch Neurol 2009;

66(10): 1210-5.
[http://dx.doi.org/10.1001/archneurol.2009.201] [PMID: 19822776]

[77] Anstey KJ, Mack HA, Cherbuin N. Alcohol consumption as a risk factor for dementia and cognitive decline: meta-analysis of prospective studies. Am J Geriatr Psychiatry 2009; 17(7): 542-55. [http://dx.doi.org/10.1097/JGP.0b013e3181a2fd07] [PMID: 19546653]

[78] Lee Y, Back JH, Kim J, *et al.* Systematic review of health behavioral risks and cognitive health in older adults. Int Psychogeriatr 2010; 22(2): 174-87. [http://dx.doi.org/10.1017/S1041610209991189] [PMID: 19883522]

[79] Singh B, Parsaik AK, Mielke MM, *et al.* Association of Mediterranean diet with mild cognitive impairment and Alzheimer's disease: a systematic review and meta-analysis. J Alzheimers Dis 2014; 39(2): 271-82. [PMID: 24164735]

CHAPTER 6

New Horizons in Ischaemic Stroke among Older People

Tuck Yean Yong[1,*], Kareeann Sok Fun Khow[2]

[1] *Internal Medicine, Flinders Private Hospital, Flinders Drive, Bedford Park, South Australia 5042, Australia*

[2] *Aged and Extended Care Services, The Queen Elizabeth Hospital and Department of Medicine, University of Adelaide, Adelaide, South Australia, Australia*

Abstract: The incidence and prevalence of ischaemic stroke increase substantially with age. In addition, clinical outcomes after a stroke are influenced significantly by age. Risk factor profiles for ischaemic stroke differ between young and older patients. Furthermore older patients with ischaemic stroke often receive less effective treatment and experience poorer outcomes than the younger population. For those who survive an acute ischaemic stroke, a comprehensive approach involving lifestyle modifications, antiplatelet or anticoagulant therapy, blood-pressure control, cholesterol-lowering and carotid artery stenosis intervention where applicable, is effective in reducing the risk of recurrent stroke. Long-term rehabilitation and supportive care is critical in the management of older people after an acute ischaemic stroke. Future research is still needed to reduce the incidence of ischaemic stroke and improve outcomes in the older population..

Keywords: Anticoagulant, Antiplatelet therapy, Carotid artery stenosis, Hypertension, Older, Rehabilitation, Risk factors, Secondary prevention, Stroke.

INTRODUCTION

Worldwide, about 16 million first episode of stroke occur annually and 5.7 million die from it each year [1]. Stroke is the second most common cause of death after

* **Correspondence author Tuck Yean Yong:** Internal Medicine, Flinders Private Hospital, Flinders Drive, Bedford Park, South Australia 5042, Australia; Tel: +61 8 8241 2121; Fax: +61 8 8240 0879; E-mail: tyyong@hotmail.com.

Tuck Yean Yong (Ed)

myocardial infarction [1] and is associated with one of the highest rates of disability in adults [2]. Up to 50% of stroke survivors were unable to regain independence and need long-term personal care [3]. Stroke can affect individual of any age but the incidence and prevalence increase significantly with advancing age [4]. For each successive decade after the age of 55 years, the rate of stroke doubles in both men and women [5]. With an aging population, the incidence and economic burden of ischaemic stroke is expected to rise.

Patients with stroke are at increased risk for further vascular events including recurrent ischaemic stroke (highest risk), acute myocardial infarction and death from other vascular causes. The risk of recurrent stroke is highest in the early period after an acute event and therefore, secondary prevention strategies are essential [6]. Older people who survive an acute ischaemic stroke often need long-term rehabilitation and supportive care.

This chapter will examine the differences in clinical outcomes among older people who experience ischaemic stroke in comparison to the younger population and review secondary prevention strategies and rehabilitation approaches after a stroke event.

CLINICAL OUTCOMES AND EVALUATION

In comparison to younger patients, older people with strokes have more severe neurological deficits at presentation and they recover more slowly [7, 8]. Older people who survive a stroke are more likely to require assistance in activities of daily living or to need care in a residential facility compared to younger patients [9]. This difference can be explained by medical and functional status before the stroke, pre-existing multiple organ dysfunction, polypharmacy and severity of stroke [7, 10].

After the first ischaemic stroke or transient ischaemic attack (TIA), people aged >65 years have a three-fold increase in risk for a recurrence within the next 10 years compared with those below this age [11]. Increasing age has been observed to be an independent risk factor associated with mortality both in the short- and long-term after acute ischaemic stroke [12]. In several studies, the stroke mortality rate is highest among people aged 75 years and above but the reason is uncertain

[12, 13]. Several important factors may be contributory including stroke severity, higher frequency of atrial fibrillation (which is associated with higher mortality) [14] and the presence of comorbidities [10].

In the evaluation of stroke or TIA, brain imaging is mandatory for diagnosis, classification and management. Magnetic resonance imaging (MRI) is more sensitive than computed tomography (CT) in the diagnosis of acute ischaemic stroke [15] but it may not be available widely. Next, arterial imaging with the use of carotid Doppler ultrasonography, CT angiography or magnetic resonance angiography (MRA) is usually necessary. Electrocardiography (ECG) must be performed to identify if atrial fibrillation is present. Occasionally ambulatory ECG is needed to detect paroxysmal atrial fibrillation. Transthoracic or transoesophageal echocardiography is often used to identify cardiac sources of embolism other than atrial fibrillation. Blood investigations are useful to show other contributing factors such as primary erythrocytosis, hyperglycaemia, kidney dysfunction and electrolyte disturbances.

STROKE UNITS

Admission to a stroke unit has been demonstrated to benefit patients of all ages [16, 17]. Such care may enable an extra five patients out of every 100 to return home [18]. Early mobilisation and correction of abnormal physiological parameters after stroke have been shown to improve stroke care, minimize disability and complications, improve long-term survival and decrease the risk of recurrence [15, 19, 20].

SECONDARY PREVENTION

Intensive risk factor treatment and lifestyle modification are essential in all patients after an acute ischaemic stroke, regardless of age. It is estimated that at least 80% of recurrent events might be prevented with the use of a comprehensive approach that includes exercise, dietary modification, antiplatelet or anticoagulant therapy, blood pressure and cholesterol control [21]. Carotid endarectomy should be considered in selective patients [22]. Observational studies of patients with a previous stroke showed that healthy lifestyle behaviours including regular exercise and abstinence from smoking are associated with a reduced risk of mortality [23].

Antiplatelet Therapy

Through inhibition of platelet adhesion and aggregation, antiplatelet agents have an important role in primary and secondary prevention of acute ischaemic stroke. Aspirin reduces early mortality in patients after acute ischaemic strokes when administered within 48 h of symptom onset. In this setting, aspirin decreases the risk of all vascular events by about 22% [24 - 26].

Current clinical guidelines indicate that aspirin alone, clopidogrel (an adenosine disphosphate-receptor inhibitor) and the combination of aspirin and dipyridamole (a phosphodiesterase inhibitor) are all acceptable first-line options in secondary stroke prevention [22, 27]. Randomised trials for long-term secondary prevention of ischaemic stroke have not shown any significant benefit with the combination of clopidogrel and aspirin compared with either clopidogrel or aspirin monotherapy [28, 29]. Currently, limited evidence is available for the risk-benefit of combination antiplatelet therapy in the very old (age ≥85 years).

Anticoagulant Therapy and Atrial Fibrillation

Atrial fibrillation causes at least 15% of ischaemic strokes [5]. The rates of stroke and major bleeding increase with increasing age in people with atrial fibrillation. The CHA_2DS_2-VASc risk score (Table **1**) is used to assess risk of stroke in atrial fibrillation [30].

Table 1. Scoring system for evaluation of stroke risk (CHA_2DS_2-VASc) in patients with atrial fibrillation.

CHA_2DS_2-VASc	**Score**
Congestive heart failure	1
Hypertension	1
Age ≥75 years	2
Diabetes mellitus	1
Stroke/Transient ischaemic attack/Thromboembolism	2
Vascular disease (prior myocardial infarction or peripheral artery disease or aortic plaque)	1
Age 65-74 years	1

(Table 1) contd.....

CHA_2DS_2-VASc	**Score**
Sex category (*i.e.*, female sex)	1
Maximum Score	**9**

The score includes two points for age ≥75 years, one point for age 65-74 years and two points for previous stroke, TIA or thromboembolism. Therefore oral anticoagulation is indicated in almost all older patients with atrial fibrillation after a stroke or TIA.

In patients with atrial fibrillation, dose-adjusted warfarin (a vitamin K antagonist) decreases the risk of ischaemic stroke by 68% with no significant increase in major bleeding (Table **2**) [31, 32]. In the subgroup analysis of patients aged >75 years, warfarin reduced stroke risk and the efficacy was consistent across all studies. In patients aged >75 years with atrial fibrillation, studies have shown that warfarin is effective and safe in reducing both recurrent thromboembolic strokes and mortality [33, 34]. However, warfarin use necessitate regular monitoring of the international normalized ratio (INR) of antithrombin time and avoidance of drug interactions which can be challenging in older people on multiple medications.

Table 2. Results of key trials for secondary prevention of stroke.

Strategy	**Study**	**Primary End Points**	**Results***
Antiplatelet therapy			
Aspirin	ATTC: aspirin *vs.* placebo	Nonfatal stroke, nonfatal MI and death from vascular causes	RRR: 13.0% ARR: 1.0% NNT: 100†
Clopidogrel	CAPRIE: clopidogrel *vs.* aspirin	Ischaemic stroke, MI and death from vascular causes	RRR: 8.7% ARR: 0.5% NNT: 196
Aspirin and dipyridamole	ESPS2: aspirin and dipyridamole *vs.* aspirin	Stroke	RRR: 23.8% ARR: 3.0% NNT: 74
Anticogulation in atrial fibrillation			
Warfarin	EAFT: warfarin *vs* placebo	All strokes	RRR: 66.0% ARR: 8.0% NNT: 12

(Table 2) contd.....

Strategy	Study	Primary End Points	Results*
Dabigatran	*vs.* warfarin	Stroke and systemic embolism	RRR: 34.0% ARR: 0.6% NNT: 172‡
Rivaroxaban	ROCKET AF: rivaroxaban *vs.* warfarin	Stroke and systemic embolism	RRR: 13.0% ARR: 0.3% NNT: 333
Apixaban	ARISTOTLE: apixaban *vs.* warfarin	Stroke and systemic embolism	RRR: 21.0% ARR: 0.3% NNT: 303
Blood-pressure control	PROGRESS: ACE inhibitor + diuretic *vs.* placebo	Total strokes	RRR: 28.0% ARR: 4.0% NNT: 97
Carotid endarectomy (for symptomatic high grade stenosis)	NASCET: carotid endarectomy + medical treatment *vs.* medical treatment alone	Any ipsilateral ischaemic stroke	RRR: 65.0% ARR: 17.0% NNT: 9

*The relative risk reduction (RRR) and absolute risk reduction (ARR) are annualized for all the studies except ESPS2, NASCET and PROGRESS, for which the RRR and ARR are for the duration of the trial. The number needed to treat (NNT) to prevent one primary-outcome event (secondary prevention) per year was calculated with the data on ARR.

†The results are based on a meta-analysis of trials comparing aspirin with placebo in patients with a previous stroke or transient ischaemic attack

‡The results are based on dabigatran at a dose of 150 mg twice a day

ACE: Angiotensin-converting enzyme, ARISTOTLE: Apixaban for Reduction in Stroke and Other Thromboembolic Events in Atrial Fibrillation, ATTC: Antithrombotic Trialists' Collaboration, CAPRIE: Clopidogrel *versus* Aspirin in Patients at Risk of Ischemic Events, EAFT: European Atrial Fibrillation Trial, ESPS2: European Stroke Prevention Study 2, MI: Myocardial infarction, NASCET: North American Symptomatic Carotid Endaterectomy Trial, PROGRESS: Perindopril Protection against Recurrent Stroke Study, RE-LY: Randomized Evaluation of Long-Term Anticogulation Therapy, ROCKET AF: Rivaroxaban Once Daily Oral Direct Factor Xa Inhibition Compared with Vitamin K Antagonism for Prevention of Stroke and Embolism Trial in Atrial Fibrillation.

Newer oral anticoagulants are now available which do not require INR monitoring and have replaced warfarin in some cases. In a randomised trial of participants with atrial fibrillation (20% had a prior stroke or TIA), dabigatran (a direct thrombin inhibitor) at a dose of 150 mg twice a day, was superior to warfarin in the prevention of ischaemic stroke or systemic embolism, with a comparable rate of major bleeding but a significantly lower risk of intracranial haemorrhage [35]. At a lower dose of 110 mg twice a day, dabigatran was non-inferior to warfarin with a reduced risk of major bleeding. With dabigatran, there is a significant interaction between age and increased risk of bleeding in older people compared with younger patients [36]. The European Society of Cardiology recommends the lower dose of dabigatran (110 mg twice a day) for patients aged ≥80 years [37]. Because dabigatran is cleared by the kidneys, dose should be lowered to 110 mg twice a day when creatinine clearance is <50 mL/min and contraindicated if creatinine clearance is <30 mL/min. Since creatinine clearance diminishes over time with ageing, regular checks of the kidney function should be performed in older patients [38].

Randomized trials have also shown factor Xa inhibitors are effective in reducing the risk of stroke among patients with atrial fibrillation. Apixaban has been found to be superior to warfarin, with reductions in the risk of mortality and bleeding [39]. With apixaban, patients aged ≥75 years consistently had less bleeding than those on warfarin [40]. If two of these three factors (age ≥80 years, body weight ≤60 kg or serum creatinine ≥133 µmol/L [1.5 mg/dL]) are present, the dose of apixaban should be halved (2.5 mg twice a day) [38]. Rivaroxaban was non-inferior to warfarin, with a lower risk of bleeding [41]. In patients with creatinine clearance of <50 mL/min, rivaroxaban dose should be reduced to 15 mg once a day, 25% lower than standard dose [38].

Blood Pressure Control

Blood pressure is the most important risk factor in both primary and secondary prevention of stroke. Across all age groups, studies of blood pressure reduction have demonstrated a reduction of 30-40% reduction of stroke incidence [42]. In the Hypertension in the Very Elderly Trial (HYVET) which studied the treatment of hypertension using indapamide with or without perindopril in people aged ≥80 years, demonstrated a 39% reduction in the rate of fatal or nonfatal stroke, a 39% reduction in stroke-related death and a 21% reduction in all-cause mortality [43]. Antihypertensive treatment has also been found to reduce the risk of recurrent ischaemic stroke by about 30% (Table **2**) [44 - 46].

Cholesterol-Lowering Treatment

Lowering cholesterol levels with statin drugs has been proven effective in secondary prevention after stroke or TIA. The Stroke Prevention by Aggressive Reduction in Cholesterol Levels (SPARCL), a placebo-controlled trial demonstrated that atorvastatin reduced the risk of recurrent stroke in both the older and young patient groups compared with controls [47]. A meta-analysis also revealed that statins in reduced all-cause mortality and stroke by 25% in older patients as part of secondary prevention [48].

Carotid Artery Stenosis Treatment

Carotid artery stenosis is one of the major risk factor for ischaemic stroke [49]. Despite a high incidence of carotid artery stenosis in older people [50], such stenosis is substantially under investigated in patients with stroke or TIA who are aged ≥80 years [51]. Carotid endarterectomy is indicated for treatment of patients with a history of non-disabling ischaemic stroke or TIA who have high grade (70-99%) carotid stenosis or, in selected cases, moderate (50-69%) stenosis [52]. Older patients can safely and successfully undergo carotid endarterectomy with recurrent stroke and mortality rates similar between the young (aged <65 years) and older (aged 65-79 years) groups [53, 54]. In terms of the timing of carotid endarterectomy after an ischaemic stroke or TIA, early intervention within 2 weeks after the onset of symptoms, is now recommended, given that benefits of surgery rapidly diminish with increasing time after the event [55].

Compared to carotid endarterectomy, stenting is less invasive and associated with a faster recovery and a lower risk of cranial-nerve palsies [56]. However, studies have found that the periprocedural risk of death and recurrent stroke within 30 days are significantly higher with carotid-artery stenting than with endarterectomy [56, 57]. Findings from Carotid Revascularization Endarterectomy *versus* Stenting Trial (CREST) and European stenting trials have demonstrated that the relative benefits and risks of these procedures differ with age [56, 58]. In patients older than 70 years, carotid endarterectomy have been found to be superior to carotid-artery stenting, whereas in patients 70 years or younger, the periprocedural risks of stroke and death are similar in both procedures.

REHABILITATION

Older patients who survive a stroke event often need long-term rehabilitation and supportive care. Rehabilitation of older people after ischaemic stroke generally relies on the training of patients in compensatory strategies [59]. Improved motor control can be achieved with task-specific training that incorporates increased use of proximal and distal movements during intensive practice of real-world activities [60]. The amount of practice correlates with gains for a given level of residual movement ability. Patients should be encouraged to gradually build greater strength, speed, endurance, and precision of multi-joint movements on tasks that are important for independence and daily activity [61, 62].

CONCLUSION

The incidence of stroke and rates of adverse outcome after stroke increase with age. With the growing elderly population, the prevalence of stroke is expected to rise. Older patients with ischaemic stroke often receive less effective treatment and have poorer outcomes than younger ones. Current long-term management after an acute ischaemic stroke in older people is focused on secondary prevention or recurrent stroke and rehabilitation. Future research is needed to consider age as a factor that influences stroke prevention and treatment so that the incidence can be reduced and outcomes improved in this vulnerable group.

CONFLICT OF INTEREST

The author confirms that author has no conflict of interest to declare for this publication.

ACKNOWLEDGEMENTS

Declared none.

KEY POINTS

- Over 80% of ischaemic strokes occur in older people aged ≥65 years.
- Clinical outcomes after an acute ischaemic stroke are highly affected by age.
- Secondary prevention of strokes in older people should include abstinence from smoking, antiplatelet or anticoagulant therapy, blood pressure control, cholesterol-lowering and carotid artery stenosis treatment where indicated.
- Older patients who survive an ischaemic stroke often need long-term rehabilitation and supportive care.

REFERENCES

[1] Strong K, Mathers C, Bonita R. Preventing stroke: saving lives around the world. Lancet Neurol 2007; 6(2): 182-7.
[http://dx.doi.org/10.1016/S1474-4422(07)70031-5] [PMID: 17239805]

[2] Hendricks HT, van Limbeek J, Geurts AC, Zwarts MJ. Motor recovery after stroke: a systematic review of the literature. Arch Phys Med Rehabil 2002; 83(11): 1629-37.
[http://dx.doi.org/10.1053/apmr.2002.35473] [PMID: 12422337]

[3] Sturm JW, Donnan GA, Dewey HM, *et al.* Quality of life after stroke: the North East Melbourne Stroke Incidence Study (NEMESIS). Stroke 2004; 35(10): 2340-5.
[http://dx.doi.org/10.1161/01.STR.0000141977.18520.3b] [PMID: 15331799]

[4] Goldstein LB, Adams R, Alberts MJ, *et al.* Primary prevention of ischemic stroke: a guideline from the American Heart Association/American Stroke Association Stroke Council: cosponsored by the Atherosclerotic Peripheral Vascular Disease Interdisciplinary Working Group; Cardiovascular Nursing Council; Clinical Cardiology Council; Nutrition, Physical Activity, and Metabolism Council; and the Quality of Care and Outcomes Research Interdisciplinary Working Group: the American Academy of Neurology affirms the value of this guideline. Stroke 2006; 37(6): 1583-633.
[http://dx.doi.org/10.1161/01.STR.0000223048.70103.F1] [PMID: 16675728]

[5] Rojas JI, Zurrú MC, Romano M, Patrucco L, Cristiano E. Acute ischemic stroke and transient ischemic attack in the very old--risk factor profile and stroke subtype between patients older than 80 years and patients aged less than 80 years. Eur J Neurol 2007; 14(8): 895-9.
[http://dx.doi.org/10.1111/j.1468-1331.2007.01841.x] [PMID: 17662011]

[6] Giles MF, Rothwell PM. Risk of stroke early after transient ischaemic attack: a systematic review and meta-analysis. Lancet Neurol 2007; 6(12): 1063-72.
[http://dx.doi.org/10.1016/S1474-4422(07)70274-0] [PMID: 17993293]

[7] Kammersgaard LP, Jørgensen HS, Reith J, Nakayama H, Pedersen PM, Olsen TS. Short- and long-term prognosis for very old stroke patients. The Copenhagen Stroke Study. Age Ageing 2004; 33(2): 149-54.
[http://dx.doi.org/10.1093/ageing/afh052] [PMID: 14960430]

[8] Marini C, Baldassarre M, Russo T, *et al.* Burden of first-ever ischemic stroke in the oldest old: evidence from a population-based study. Neurology 2004; 62(1): 77-81.
[http://dx.doi.org/10.1212/01.WNL.0000101461.61501.65] [PMID: 14718701]

[9] Hankey GJ, Jamrozik K, Broadhurst RJ, Forbes S, Anderson CS. Long-term disability after first-ever stroke and related prognostic factors in the Perth Community Stroke Study, 1989-1990. Stroke 2002; 33(4): 1034-40.
[http://dx.doi.org/10.1161/01.STR.0000012515.66889.24] [PMID: 11935057]

[10] Di Carlo A, Baldereschi M, Gandolfo C, *et al.* Stroke in an elderly population: incidence and impact on survival and daily function. Cerebrovasc Dis 2003; 16(2): 141-50.
[http://dx.doi.org/10.1159/000070594] [PMID: 12792172]

[11] Fonarow GC, Reeves MJ, Zhao X, *et al.* Age-related differences in characteristics, performance measures, treatment trends, and outcomes in patients with ischemic stroke. Circulation 2010; 121(7): 879-91.

[http://dx.doi.org/10.1161/CIRCULATIONAHA.109.892497] [PMID: 20142445]

[12] Collins TC, Petersen NJ, Menke TJ, Souchek J, Foster W, Ashton CM. Short-term, intermediate-term, and long-term mortality in patients hospitalized for stroke. J Clin Epidemiol 2003; 56(1): 81-7. [http://dx.doi.org/10.1016/S0895-4356(02)00570-X] [PMID: 12589874]

[13] Carter AM, Catto AJ, Mansfield MW, Bamford JM, Grant PJ. Predictive variables for mortality after acute ischemic stroke. Stroke 2007; 38(6): 1873-80. [http://dx.doi.org/10.1161/STROKEAHA.106.474569] [PMID: 17446429]

[14] Steger C, Pratter A, Martinek-Bregel M, *et al.* Stroke patients with atrial fibrillation have a worse prognosis than patients without: data from the Austrian Stroke registry. Eur Heart J 2004; 25(19): 1734-40. [http://dx.doi.org/10.1016/j.ehj.2004.06.030] [PMID: 15451152]

[15] Jauch EC, Saver JL, Adams HP Jr, *et al.* Guidelines for the early management of patients with acute ischemic stroke: a guideline for healthcare professionals from the American Heart Association/American Stroke Association. Stroke 2013; 44(3): 870-947. [http://dx.doi.org/10.1161/STR.0b013e318284056a] [PMID: 23370205]

[16] Candelise L, Gattinoni M, Bersano A, Micieli G, Sterzi R, Morabito A. Stroke-unit care for acute stroke patients: an observational follow-up study. Lancet 2007; 369(9558): 299-305. [http://dx.doi.org/10.1016/S0140-6736(07)60152-4] [PMID: 17258670]

[17] Saposnik G, Kapral MK, Coutts SB, Fang J, Demchuk AM, Hill MD. Do all age groups benefit from organized inpatient stroke care? Stroke 2009; 40(10): 3321-7. [http://dx.doi.org/10.1161/STROKEAHA.109.554907] [PMID: 19644068]

[18] Langhorne P, Duncan P. Does the organization of postacute stroke care really matter? Stroke 2001; 32(1): 268-74. [http://dx.doi.org/10.1161/01.STR.32.1.268] [PMID: 11136947]

[19] The impact of standardized stroke orders on adherence to best practices. Neurology 2005; 65(3): 360-5. [http://dx.doi.org/10.1212/01.wnl.0000171706.68756.b7] [PMID: 16087898]

[20] Organised inpatient (stroke unit) care for stroke. Cochrane Database Syst Rev 2013; 9: CD000197. [PMID: 24026639]

[21] Hackam DG, Spence JD. Combining multiple approaches for the secondary prevention of vascular events after stroke: a quantitative modeling study. Stroke 2007; 38(6): 1881-5. [http://dx.doi.org/10.1161/STROKEAHA.106.475525] [PMID: 17431209]

[22] Furie KL, Kasner SE, Adams RJ, *et al.* Guidelines for the prevention of stroke in patients with stroke or transient ischemic attack: a guideline for healthcare professionals from the American heart association/American stroke association. Stroke 2011; 42(1): 227-76. [http://dx.doi.org/10.1161/STR.0b013e3181f7d043] [PMID: 20966421]

[23] Towfighi A, Markovic D, Ovbiagele B. Impact of a healthy lifestyle on all-cause and cardiovascular mortality after stroke in the USA. J Neurol Neurosurg Psychiatry 2012; 83(2): 146-51. [http://dx.doi.org/10.1136/jnnp-2011-300743] [PMID: 22019548]

[24] CAST: randomised placebo-controlled trial of early aspirin use in 20,000 patients with acute ischaemic

stroke. Lancet 1997; 349(9066): 1641-9.
[http://dx.doi.org/10.1016/S0140-6736(97)04010-5] [PMID: 9186381]

[25] Collaborative overview of randomised trials of antiplatelet therapy--I: Prevention of death, myocardial infarction, and stroke by prolonged antiplatelet therapy in various categories of patients. Antiplatelet Trialists' Collaboration. BMJ 1994; 308(6921): 81-106.
[http://dx.doi.org/10.1136/bmj.308.6921.81] [PMID: 8298418]

[26] The International Stroke Trial (IST): a randomised trial of aspirin, subcutaneous heparin, both, or neither among 19435 patients with acute ischaemic stroke. Lancet 1997; 349(9065): 1569-81.
[http://dx.doi.org/10.1016/S0140-6736(97)04011-7] [PMID: 9174558]

[27] Diener HC, Cunha L, Forbes C, Sivenius J, Smets P, Lowenthal A. European Stroke Prevention Study. 2. Dipyridamole and acetylsalicylic acid in the secondary prevention of stroke. J Neurol Sci 1996; 143(1-2): 1-13.
[http://dx.doi.org/10.1016/S0022-510X(96)00308-5] [PMID: 8981292]

[28] Diener HC, Bogousslavsky J, Brass LM, *et al.* Aspirin and clopidogrel compared with clopidogrel alone after recent ischaemic stroke or transient ischaemic attack in high-risk patients (MATCH): randomised, double-blind, placebo-controlled trial. Lancet 2004; 364(9431): 331-7.
[http://dx.doi.org/10.1016/S0140-6736(04)16721-4] [PMID: 15276392]

[29] Bhatt DL, Fox KA, Hacke W, *et al.* Clopidogrel and aspirin *versus* aspirin alone for the prevention of atherothrombotic events. N Engl J Med 2006; 354(16): 1706-17.
[http://dx.doi.org/10.1056/NEJMoa060989] [PMID: 16531616]

[30] Lane DA, Lip GY. Use of the CHA(2)DS(2)-VASc and HAS-BLED scores to aid decision making for thromboprophylaxis in non-valvular atrial fibrillation. Circulation 2012; 126(7): 860-5.
[http://dx.doi.org/10.1161/CIRCULATIONAHA.111.060061] [PMID: 22891166]

[31] Risk factors for stroke and efficacy of antithrombotic therapy in atrial fibrillation. Analysis of pooled data from five randomized controlled trials. Arch Intern Med 1994; 154(13): 1449-57.
[http://dx.doi.org/10.1001/archinte.1994.00420130036007] [PMID: 8018000]

[32] Secondary prevention in non-rheumatic atrial fibrillation after transient ischaemic attack or minor stroke. Lancet 1993; 342(8882): 1255-62.
[PMID: 7901582]

[33] Mant J, Hobbs FD, Fletcher K, *et al.* Warfarin *versus* aspirin for stroke prevention in an elderly community population with atrial fibrillation (the Birmingham Atrial Fibrillation Treatment of the Aged Study, BAFTA): a randomised controlled trial. Lancet 2007; 370(9586): 493-503.
[http://dx.doi.org/10.1016/S0140-6736(07)61233-1] [PMID: 17693178]

[34] Tsivgoulis G, Spengos K, Zakopoulos N, Manios E, Peppes V, Vemmos K. Efficacy of anticoagulation for secondary stroke prevention in older people with non-valvular atrial fibrillation: a prospective case series study. Age Ageing 2005; 34(1): 35-40.
[http://dx.doi.org/10.1093/ageing/afi004] [PMID: 15591481]

[35] Connolly SJ, Ezekowitz MD, Yusuf S, *et al.* Dabigatran *versus* warfarin in patients with atrial fibrillation. N Engl J Med 2009; 361(12): 1139-51.
[http://dx.doi.org/10.1056/NEJMoa0905561] [PMID: 19717844]

[36] Eikelboom JW, Wallentin L, Connolly SJ, *et al.* Risk of bleeding with 2 doses of dabigatran compared with warfarin in older and younger patients with atrial fibrillation: an analysis of the randomized evaluation of long-term anticoagulant therapy (RE-LY) trial. Circulation 2011; 123(21): 2363-72. [http://dx.doi.org/10.1161/CIRCULATIONAHA.110.004747] [PMID: 21576658]

[37] Camm AJ, Lip GY, De Caterina R, *et al.* 2012 focused update of the ESC Guidelines for the management of atrial fibrillation: an update of the 2010 ESC Guidelines for the management of atrial fibrillation. Developed with the special contribution of the European Heart Rhythm Association. Eur Heart J 2012; 33(21): 2719-47. [http://dx.doi.org/10.1093/eurheartj/ehs253] [PMID: 22922413]

[38] Heidbuchel H, Verhamme P, Alings M, *et al.* European Heart Rhythm Association Practical Guide on the use of new oral anticoagulants in patients with non-valvular atrial fibrillation. Europace 2013; 15(5): 625-51. [http://dx.doi.org/10.1093/europace/eut083] [PMID: 23625942]

[39] Granger CB, Alexander JH, McMurray JJ, *et al.* Apixaban *versus* warfarin in patients with atrial fibrillation. N Engl J Med 2011; 365(11): 981-92. [http://dx.doi.org/10.1056/NEJMoa1107039] [PMID: 21870978]

[40] Halvorsen S, Atar D, Yang H, *et al.* Efficacy and safety of apixaban compared with warfarin according to age for stroke prevention in atrial fibrillation: observations from the ARISTOTLE trial. Eur Heart J 2014; 35(28): 1864-72. [http://dx.doi.org/10.1093/eurheartj/ehu046] [PMID: 24561548]

[41] Patel MR, Mahaffey KW, Garg J, *et al.* Rivaroxaban *versus* warfarin in nonvalvular atrial fibrillation. N Engl J Med 2011; 365(10): 883-91. [http://dx.doi.org/10.1056/NEJMoa1009638] [PMID: 21830957]

[42] Turnbull F, Neal B, Ninomiya T, *et al.* Effects of different regimens to lower blood pressure on major cardiovascular events in older and younger adults: meta-analysis of randomised trials. BMJ 2008; 336(7653): 1121-3. [http://dx.doi.org/10.1136/bmj.39548.738368.BE] [PMID: 18480116]

[43] Beckett NS, Peters R, Fletcher AE, *et al.* Treatment of hypertension in patients 80 years of age or older. N Engl J Med 2008; 358(18): 1887-98. [http://dx.doi.org/10.1056/NEJMoa0801369] [PMID: 18378519]

[44] Chalmers J, Todd A, Chapman N, *et al.* International Society of Hypertension (ISH): statement on blood pressure lowering and stroke prevention. J Hypertens 2003; 21(4): 651-63. [http://dx.doi.org/10.1097/00004872-200304000-00001] [PMID: 12658005]

[45] Prevention of stroke by antihypertensive drug treatment in older persons with isolated systolic hypertension. Final results of the Systolic Hypertension in the Elderly Program (SHEP). JAMA 1991; 265(24): 3255-64. [http://dx.doi.org/10.1001/jama.1991.03460240051027] [PMID: 2046107]

[46] Randomised trial of a perindopril-based blood-pressure-lowering regimen among 6,105 individuals with previous stroke or transient ischaemic attack. Lancet 2001; 358(9287): 1033-41. [http://dx.doi.org/10.1016/S0140-6736(01)06178-5] [PMID: 11589932]

[47] Chaturvedi S, Zivin J, Breazna A, *et al.* Effect of atorvastatin in elderly patients with a recent stroke or transient ischemic attack. Neurology 2009; 72(8): 688-94. [http://dx.doi.org/10.1212/01.wnl.0000327339.55844.1a] [PMID: 18768917]

[48] Afilalo J, Duque G, Steele R, Jukema JW, de Craen AJ, Eisenberg MJ. Statins for secondary prevention in elderly patients: a hierarchical bayesian meta-analysis. J Am Coll Cardiol 2008; 51(1): 37-45. [http://dx.doi.org/10.1016/j.jacc.2007.06.063] [PMID: 18174034]

[49] Chaturvedi S, Matsumura JS, Gray W, Xu C, Verta P. Carotid artery stenting in octogenarians: periprocedural stroke risk predictor analysis from the multicenter Carotid ACCULINK/ACCUNET Post Approval Trial to Uncover Rare Events (CAPTURE 2) clinical trial. Stroke 2010; 41(4): 757-64. [http://dx.doi.org/10.1161/STROKEAHA.109.569426] [PMID: 20185789]

[50] de Weerd M, Greving JP, de Jong AW, Buskens E, Bots ML. Prevalence of asymptomatic carotid artery stenosis according to age and sex: systematic review and metaregression analysis. Stroke 2009; 40(4): 1105-13. [http://dx.doi.org/10.1161/STROKEAHA.108.532218] [PMID: 19246704]

[51] Fairhead JF, Rothwell PM. Under investigation and undertreatment of carotid disease in elderly patients with transient ischaemic attack and stroke: comparative population based study. BMJ 2006; 333(7567): 525-7. [http://dx.doi.org/10.1136/bmj.38895.646898.55] [PMID: 16849366]

[52] Guidelines for management of ischaemic stroke and transient ischaemic attack 2008. Cerebrovasc Dis 2008; 25(5): 457-507. [http://dx.doi.org/10.1159/000131083] [PMID: 18477843]

[53] Miller MT, Comerota AJ, Tzilinis A, Daoud Y, Hammerling J. Carotid endarterectomy in octogenarians: does increased age indicate "high risk?". J Vasc Surg 2005; 41(2): 231-7. [http://dx.doi.org/10.1016/j.jvs.2004.11.021] [PMID: 15768004]

[54] Teso D, Edwards RE, Frattini JC, Dudrick SJ, Dardik A. Safety of carotid endarterectomy in 2,443 elderly patients: lessons from nonagenarians--are we pushing the limit? J Am Coll Surg 2005; 200(5): 734-41. [http://dx.doi.org/10.1016/j.jamcollsurg.2004.12.012] [PMID: 15848366]

[55] Rothwell PM, Eliasziw M, Gutnikov SA, Warlow CP, Barnett HJ. Endarterectomy for symptomatic carotid stenosis in relation to clinical subgroups and timing of surgery. Lancet 2004; 363(9413): 915-24. [http://dx.doi.org/10.1016/S0140-6736(04)15785-1] [PMID: 15043958]

[56] Brott TG, Hobson RW II, Howard G, *et al.* Stenting *versus* endarterectomy for treatment of carotid-artery stenosis. N Engl J Med 2010; 363(1): 11-23. [http://dx.doi.org/10.1056/NEJMoa0912321] [PMID: 20505173]

[57] Ederle J, Dobson J, Featherstone RL, *et al.* Carotid artery stenting compared with endarterectomy in patients with symptomatic carotid stenosis (International Carotid Stenting Study): an interim analysis of a randomised controlled trial. Lancet 2010; 375(9719): 985-97. [http://dx.doi.org/10.1016/S0140-6736(10)60239-5] [PMID: 20189239]

[58] Bonati LH, Dobson J, Algra A, *et al.* Short-term outcome after stenting *versus* endarterectomy for symptomatic carotid stenosis: a preplanned meta-analysis of individual patient data. Lancet 2010; 376(9746): 1062-73.
[http://dx.doi.org/10.1016/S0140-6736(10)61009-4] [PMID: 20832852]

[59] Dobkin BH. Strategies for stroke rehabilitation. Lancet Neurol 2004; 3(9): 528-36.
[http://dx.doi.org/10.1016/S1474-4422(04)00851-8] [PMID: 15324721]

[60] Kwakkel G, van Peppen R, Wagenaar RC, *et al.* Effects of augmented exercise therapy time after stroke: a meta-analysis. Stroke 2004; 35(11): 2529-39.
[http://dx.doi.org/10.1161/01.STR.0000143153.76460.7d] [PMID: 15472114]

[61] Patten C, Lexell J, Brown HE. Weakness and strength training in persons with poststroke hemiplegia: rationale, method, and efficacy. J Rehabil Res Dev 2004; 41(3A): 293-312.
[http://dx.doi.org/10.1682/JRRD.2004.03.0293] [PMID: 15543447]

[62] Saunders DH, Sanderson M, Brazzelli M, Greig CA, Mead GE. Physical fitness training for stroke patients. Cochrane Database Syst Rev 2013; 10: CD003316.
[PMID: 24142492]

CHAPTER 7

Chronic Obstructive Pulmonary Disease in Older People: Breathing Deeper with Age

Tuck Yean Yong*

Internal Medicine, Flinders Private Hospital, Flinders Drive, Bedford Park, South Australia, Australia

Abstract: Chronic obstructive pulmonary disease (COPD) is one of the most common chronic diseases in older people. COPD in the older population is a challenging disorder to diagnose and manage because of several unique age-related aspects. Age-related changes in pulmonary function can predispose older people to increased risk of mortality and other complications from COPD. The established Global Initiative for Obstructive Lung Disease criteria can be applied effectively to older people with COPD. This approach requires the use of spirometry which can be performed satisfactorily in most older patients. Treatments that are effective to reduce acute respiratory exacerbations include smoking cessation, vaccinations against influenza and pneumococcus, and the use of short- and long-acting bronchodilators. Other beneficial management strategies for COPD in older adults include pulmonary rehabilitation, domiciliary oxygen and noninvasive positive airway pressure when indicated. Care should also be focused on common comorbidities associated with COPD as these can often complicate the health of older people.

Keywords: Bronchodilators, Chronic obstructive pulmonary disease, Comorbidities, Corticosteroids, Diagnosis, Domiciliary oxygen, Management, Older, Palliative care, Pulmonary rehabilitation, Smoking cessation, Spirometry.

INTRODUCTION

Chronic obstructive pulmonary disease (COPD) is a common chronic disease in

* **Correspondence author Tuck Yean Yong:** Internal Medicine, Flinders Private Hospital, Flinders Drive, Bedford Park, South Australia 5042, Australia; Tel: +61 8 8241 2121; Fax: +61 8 8240 0879; E-mail: tyyong@hotmail.com.

Tuck Yean Yong (Ed)

older people, affecting about 14% of those aged 65 years and above [1]. It is responsible for about 20% of hospital admissions of people aged 65 to 75 years [2]. COPD is associated with significant morbidity and ranks as the fourth leading cause of death worldwide. Although the burden of COPD is increasing in older people, underdiagnosis and undertreatment in this age group remain a frequent problem [3].

This chapter will focus on the diagnosis, management and prevention of COPD particularly aspects that are relevant to older adults. It will also look at the need to manage common comorbidities that are present in older patients with COPD.

AGE-RELATED CHANGES IN RESPIRATORY SYSTEM

Peak pulmonary function is usually approached at about the age of 20 years. After that, airflow limitation increases with age because of decline in lung elastic recoil, chest wall stiffness and respiratory muscle weakness [4]. Lung elastic recoil is influenced by collagen and elastin. Loss of elastic recoil with age is related to increased cross-linking of collagen and degeneration of elastin [5]. Furthermore bronchiolar airway size generally decreases after the age of 40 years irrespective of lung disease [5]. Other lung changes with increasing age include larger diameter of the alveolar ducts, smaller alveolar sacs and increase in alveolar basal laminae [5]. The overall changes of this airway pattern will lead to "senile emphysema" which can occur in non-smokers and still resemble smoking-related COPD. These age-related changes are different from airflow limitation caused by COPD, which is largely a consequence of parenchymal destruction and small airway disease.

COPD is characterised by the progressive airflow limitation, worsening slowly over years. The forced expiratory volume in 1 second/forced vital capacity (FEV_1/FVC) declines with age. On the other hand, residual volume (RV) increases with age. However there is no correlation between age and total lung capacity (TLC).

Ageing also lead to reduced chest wall compliance [4]. The loss of chest wall compliance can be a result of kyphoscoliosis, calcification of intercostal cartilage and arthritis of costovertebral joints. Moreover there are decreases in lateral intercostal muscle and diaphragm strength in older people compared to younger ones [4].

Of concern, older people have decreased perception of increases in airway resistance and less peripheral sensitivity to carbon dioxide [4]. The latter can lead to an impaired ventilatory response if hypercapnia occurs. These changes may result in disconnection between symptoms experienced and severity of respiratory dysfunction as well as delays in seeking medical attention.

EVALUATION

Clinical features commonly associated with COPD include chronic cough, persistent sputum production, dyspnoea and risk factors such as smoking and occupation-related exposure to inhaled toxins. However clinical assessment alone in older people with COPD can be challenging.

Spirometry is an objective and essential diagnostic tool of COPD and the Global Initiative for Chronic Obstructive Lung Disease (GOLD) guidelines use spirometry measurements to determine disease severity (Table **1**) [6]. Based on these guidelines, COPD is diagnosed in the presence of FEV_1/FVC of <0.7. In one study of community-dwelling older people, 75-80% was able to perform valid spirometry [7]. However frail older adults with cognitive impairment may have difficulties performing spirometry. Spirometry should be performed only in symptomatic individuals followed by postbronchodilator measurement if airflow obstruction is detected. In older people, the GOLD spirometry criteria may lead to overdiagnosis of COPD because of the lung changes that occur normally with age, as described earlier. Up to 20% of older people may be incorrectly diagnosed with COPD if spirometry criteria alone are used without consideration of clinical manifestations [8].

Other pulmonary testing may also be useful for COPD diagnosis. Lung volumes are also related to symptom manifestation and functional limitation in COPD. Hyperinflation, measured as lung volume measurements of inspiratory capacity/total lung capacity, predicts survival better than FEV_1 in COPD [9]. A reduction in the diffusion capacity of carbon monoxide is another useful clue to the presence of COPD. A 6-min walk test is also useful to determine whether oxyhaemoglobin desaturation occurs in patients with moderate or severe COPD. Those with FEV_1 <50% should also have their arterial blood gas measured to assess for hypoxia and hypercapnia.

Table 1. Global Initiative for Obstructive Lung Disease (GOLD) criteria for chronic obstructive pulmonary disease (COPD) staging.

Stage	Post-Bronchodilator FEV_1/FVC	FEV_1
I (mild)	<70% of predicted	≥80% of predicted
II (moderate)	<70% of predicted	50-79% of predicted
III (severe)	<70% of predicted	30-49% of predicted
IV (very severe)	<70% of predicted	<30% of predicted or <50% of predicted plus chronic respiratory failure

Chronic respiratory failure is defined as partial pressure of oxygen <60 mmHg (8.0 kPa) with or without partial pressure of carbon dioxide >50 mmHg (6.7 kPa) while breathing air at sea level.

COMMON COMORBIDITIES

COPD is commonly associated with several extrapulmonary comorbidities that can significantly influence a patient's quality of life and care. Examples of these comorbidities include cardiovascular diseases (CVD), osteoporosis, sarcopenia and psychiatric disorders (Table **2**) [10]. One of the mechanisms in the development of comorbid conditions in COPD is thought to be related to low-grade chronic inflammation [11].

In patients with COPD, CVD is common at rates two to three times as high as those without COPD [12, 13]. Smoking is a common risk factor for both COPD and CVD. Treatment of coronary artery disease (CAD) can be challenging. Coronary artery bypass grafting (CABG) is an effective treatment option for CAD but more adverse postoperative outcomes potentially can occur in patients with COPD because of impaired pulmonary reserve. In one study, patients with COPD aged 75 years and older receiving corticosteroids had hospital mortality of 50% with CABG [14]. This finding would suggest that alternate treatment other than CABG may be considered more appropriate for those with severe COPD aged 75 years and above. Another treatment consideration is that a small number of patients with COPD may experience bronchoconstriction if beta-blockers are used to treat CAD [15].

Table 2. Summary of common comorbidities in chronic obstructive pulmonary disease.

Comorbidity	**Prevalence**	**Clinical Impact**	**Treatment Considerations**
Cardiovascular diseases	16-53%	Decreases survival and quality of life	Cardioselective beta-blockers preferred over non-cardioselective
Osteoporosis	8-69%	Increases risk of fractures and associated disability	Minimize oral and inhaled corticosteroid use Ensure adequate vitamin D intake
Sarcopenia	15%	Decreases functional and health status	Pulmonary rehabilitation Ensure adequate vitamin D intake
Anxiety or depression	6-80%	Increases exacerbations Decreases survival and quality of life	Standard therapy for anxiety/depression Pulmonary rehabilitation Cautious use of benzodiazepines, mirtazapine and tricyclics antidepressants

In COPD, the prevalence of osteoporosis can vary between 8.4% and 69% [16, 17]. The risk of osteoporosis is increased in people with moderate-to-severe COPD compared to those without (odds ratio: 1.9%) [18]. This is particularly relevant to older people with COPD because the prevalence of osteoporosis also rises with increasing age. The presence of osteoporosis in patients with COPD has adverse prognostic implications on respiratory function, in that thoracic vertebral compression fractures are associated with pain, increased dyspnoea, worsening kyphosis, decreased vital capacity and reduced exercise tolerance [19, 20]. The identification and management of osteoporosis in COPD is similar to the general guideline.

In one study, sarcopenia affected 15% of patients with stable COPD and was associated with impaired functional and health status [21]. Sarcopenia does not impact on response to pulmonary rehabilitation, which can lead to a reversal of the syndrome in select patients [21]. There are still a limited number of studies on this association and future investigations are needed to expand the understanding of these two coexisting conditions.

Patients with COPD frequently have depressive and anxiety disorders. Depending on the study population and diagnostic definition, the prevalence of depression in

COPD has been reported between 8% and 80% [22, 23]. A meta-analysis of studies using diagnostic clinical interview showed prevalence of anxiety among patients with COPD of all ages as 10-55% in inpatients and 13-46% in outpatients [24]. One study found that about 42-46% of older people with COPD meet the diagnostic criteria for depression and anxiety disorders [25]. Anxiety or depression in patients with COPD are associated with increased hospitalizations with longer length of stay, increased mortality, decreased quality of life and reduced exercise capacity [26, 27]. Limited studies have investigated the treatment of depression or anxiety in COPD patients. At present standard therapies are employed, including cognitive behavioural therapy, antidepressants and anxiolytics [28]. However, medications such as benzodiazepines, mirtazapine and tricyclic antidepressants, can suppress the respiratory drive and should be used with caution [28]. Pulmonary rehabilitation has been demonstrated to reduce symptoms of anxiety and depression, with associated improvement in quality of life [28].

MANAGEMENT OF COPD

The core principles of COPD management include **C**ase finding and **C**onfirm diagnosis, **O**ptimise function, **P**revent deterioration, **D**evelop a care plan and manage e**X**acerbations (COPD-X) [29, 30]. Even though COPD has no cure, smoking cessation, domiciliary oxygen in hypoxaemic patients, non-invasive ventilation in selective patients and lung volume reduction surgery in people with upper lobe disease and poor exercise capacity have been found to be improve survival [31]. So far, no statistically significant improvement in survival has been observed with any of the pharmacological treatments [6]. In translating these research findings, most clinical trials on COPD therapies tend to include few older people [32].

Non-Pharmacological Interventions

Smoking Cessation

Smoking cessation is beneficial even in older people with COPD. Mortality in older adults improves with smoking cessation independent of the severity of COPD [6]. Counselling and pharmacotherapy such as nicotine replacement, bupropion and varenicline, are safe and moderately effective interventions in assisting people cease smoking [33, 34]. However, varenicline and bupropion should be used with caution due to the risk of adverse neuropsychiatric symptoms such as behavioural changes, agitation and depression [33, 34].

Physical Activity

Older people with COPD should be encouraged to engage in physical activity regularly [35]. Patients with dyspnoea have a tendency to reduce their physical activity leading to a vicious cycle of deconditioning, progressive dyspnoea with activity and further reduction in physical activity.

Nutrition

In people with COPD, low body mass index (BMI) and low fat-free mass, even in the setting of normal range BMI, independently predict mortality regardless of disease severity [36]. Careful attention should be given to nutrition status and diet as part of the management of COPD.

Pulmonary Rehabilitation

Pulmonary rehabilitation can address several aspects of COPD that are particularly important for older people such as physical deconditioning, social isolation, muscle wasting and weight loss. Pulmonary rehabilitation improves dyspnoea and health-related quality of life; and reduces duration of hospitalization in patients with COPD [37].

Pharmacological Interventions

Pharmacotherapy for COPD in older people is similar to younger ones. No treatment has been found to change the long-term decrease in lung function but can reduce symptoms and exacerbation rates, as well as improve quality of life [6]. Treatment generally includes short- and long-acting agents used in a step-wise approach according to symptom severity, pulmonary dysfunction and response to medications.

Bronchodilators

Bronchodilators, β_2-agonists and anticholinergic agents have an important role in the management of COPD. These agents can be used as monotherapy or in combination.

Beta-2 Agonists

Inhaled short-acting β_2-agonists as monotherapy are used widely for acute symptom control in COPD. Inhaled long-acting β_2-agonists, such as salmeterol and formoterol, have been shown to improve some clinical outcomes. Salmeterol improves respiratory symptoms and spirometric parameters and reduces the use of short-acting bronchodilator [38].

In older people, β_2-agonists are generally tolerated well but adverse effects such as tremor, tachycardia and hypokalaemia should be considered [32]. These agents have been associated with greater risk of arrhythmias such as supraventricular tachycardia, ventricular tachycardia, and sudden death [32]. Patients with underlying cardiac disease such as older people, are potentially more vulnerable to these arrhythmias with the use of β_2-agonists [39] but a higher mortality rate due to these complications has not been observed in several large studies [40, 41].

Anticholinergics

Ipratropium, a short-acting anticholinergic agent, has been used frequently in COPD. Ipratropium has been shown to improve lung volumes, exercise capacity and exertional dyspnoea [42]. Several long-acting anticholinergics are currently available for use in COPD. One of these long-acting anticholinergics, tiotropium, has been shown to improve dyspnoea, quality of life, FEV_1 and frequency of acute exacerbations [43]. Other new anticholinergic agents such as glycopyrronium bromide and aclidinium bromide are also available. In randomised control trials, glycopyrronium has been shown be superior to placebo and comparable with tiotropium in reducing rates of COPD exacerbation [44, 45].

The most common side-effect associated with anticholinergic agents is dry mouth. Many oral anticholinergic agents are associated with cognitive impairment but this association has not observed with the use of ipratropium in older people [46].

A meta-analysis on anticholinergic agent studies has suggested that these agents are associated with a greater risk of cardiovascular adverse events [47] but this has not been observed in a randomised controlled trial with tiotropium [43].

Inhaled Corticosteroids

In patients with moderate to severe COPD, inhaled corticosteroids (ICSs) are recommended [48] but efficacy in terms of improving FEV_1 and mortality is limited [49]. In older people, long-term high-dose ICSs should be used with caution because of the potential to cause cataracts, open-angle glaucoma, thrush and increased risk of pneumonia and bone fragility [50].

Combination Therapies

Combination therapies (long-acting β_2-agonists and ICSs) have been shown to be more effective in reducing acute exacerbations of COPD than using either agent alone [51] and demonstrated a trend towards lower mortality [40]. The combination of formoterol and tiotropium has been shown to produce improvements in airflow, hyperinflation and need for rescue therapy [52].

Several combinations of long-acting β_2-agonists and long-acting anticholinergics will be available in the near future. One study has been published on the use of a once daily fixed dose combination of both glycopyrronium (50 μg) and indacaterol (110 μg) in severe to very severe COPD [27]. This combination reduced the rate of moderate to severe exacerbations by 12% compared to glycopyrronium alone but no significant reduction was observed in comparison with open-label tiotropium. Studies involving older people have not been reported yet.

Combinations with inhaled corticosteroids, long-acting β_2-agonists and long-acting anticholinergics have also been studied in a clinical trial [51]. The triple combination (fluticasone, salmeterol and tiotropium) reduced the number of severe exacerbations requiring hospital admissions by 47%. However further studies are required to confirm the efficacy of triple therapy in older people.

Delivery Systems of Inhaled Medications

Inhaled medications can be delivered through meter-dosed inhalers, dry-powder inhaler and nebulizer. The efficacy of inhaled agents is dependent on the amount of drug delivered to the lower airways. However, older people often have difficulties using these inhalers because of arthritis, poor manual dexterity, muscle weakness, visual or cognitive impairment [53, 54].

Meter-dose inhalers have the advantage of high dose-to-dose reproducibility. However an important disadvantage of this device that should be taken into consideration in older people is the need to coordinate breathing and inhaler activation. In about 30% of older people, improper use of meter-dose inhalers can lead to a high degree of pharyngeal deposition and reduce efficacy of treatment [53]. In the same study, the use of a spacer can reduce pharyngeal deposition [53] but adherence is generally poor [55].

Dry-powder inhalers are breath-actuated and do not require coordination of inspiration and inhaler activation [56]. In one study, most older people rated the dry-powder inhaler (83% of participants) easier to use compared to metered dose inhalers (54%) [55]. However a dry-powder inhaler may require additional instructions and may prove challenging for older adults with cognitive impairment. Despite this challenges, dry-powder inhaler was still more effective than metered-dose inhaler in older people with cognitive impairment [57]. A further consideration with the use of dry-powder inhaler is the need for the patient to have a higher inspiratory flow rate, some requiring up to 30-60 L/min, compared with a minimum of 25 L/min in metered-dose inhalers [55].

Immunizations

Annual influenza vaccine is recommended for all patients with COPD. Observational studies showed that annual influenza immunization in patients with COPD reduced rates of hospitalizations for influenza and pneumonia (52% reduction), all-cause mortality and cost [58, 59]. Pneumococcal polysaccharide vaccine is recommended for all patients with COPD aged 65 years or older [6].

Surgical Interventions

Lung volume reduction surgery may be beneficial in selected patients with COPD. The best candidates for this type of surgery are those with FEV_1 >20% of predicted and a normal partial pressure of carbon dioxide or upper-lobe-predominant disease and moderate exercise tolerance [60]. Findings from the lung volume reduction surgery demonstrated higher short-term mortality (7%) but better long-term survival [61]. However, the benefits of such surgery in the older age group have not been specifically evaluated.

Other Therapies

Like younger people with severe COPD, oxygen therapy is indicated for older people if the room air resting partial oxygen pressure is <55 mmHg, or <60 mmHg in the presence of pulmonary hypertension or polycythemia. Most recommendations support more than 15 hours of use to obtain maximal benefit. Long-term oxygen therapy in these patients has been demonstrated to improve exercise ability, cognitive function and mortality [62, 63].

Theophylline is infrequently used in current practice but may be considered in patients with difficult to control COPD. However severe adverse drug events can occur with theophylline, especially in older people. Theophylline has a narrow therapeutic range of 10-20 μg/mL. It inhibits all phosphodiesterase enzyme subsets in a nonspecific way which explains the wide range of adverse effects. Older people have a higher risk of adverse drug events when taking theophylline because of concomitant diseases, reduced drug clearance and potential drug-drug interactions in the setting of polypharmacy.

New agents including combined phosphodiesterase 3 and 4 inhibitors, such as RPL554 [64], and monoclonal antibody against interleukin 1 receptor (medimmune-8986) [65] are currently under investigation for the prevention of acute exacerbations. Further work will be required to determine their efficacy in the older population.

MANAGEMENT OF ACUTE EXACERBATIONS

Severe exacerbations of COPD adversely affect health status and may cause permanent loss of lung function [66, 67]. Most of the acute exacerbations are thought to result from infections but about one-third may be of non-infectious origin [68]. A number of strategies can reduce the morbidity and mortality associated with acute exacerbations of COPD in older people.

In the treatment of exacerbations of COPD, oxygen supplementation should be titrated to achieve a target oxygen saturation range of 88-92%. This approach has been shown to have a greater than twofold reduction in mortality, compared with routine administration of high-concentration oxygen therapy [69]. This practice is equally applicable in older people with exacerbation of COPD.

Antibiotics are often used during COPD exacerbations but data is conflicting about their effectiveness. In severe COPD, effectiveness has been shown when two of these symptoms are present: increased dyspnoea, sputum volume and sputum purulence [68]. As compared with placebo, antibiotics reduce the relative risk of treatment failure (defined as no resolution or clinical deterioration) by about 50% when used during exacerbations of COPD [70].

Oral corticosteroids are useful for moderate-to-severe exacerbations of COPD. In randomized trials, treatment with prednisolone at 30-40 mg a day for 7-10 days lowered the relative risk of treatment failure (defined as intensification of therapy, rehospitalisation, or a return to the emergency department) by about 30% [71, 72]. Courses of corticosteroids extending more than 14 days do not confer any additional benefit and increase the risk of adverse events [71].

Noninvasive positive pressure ventilation, either continuous positive airway pressure or bi-level positive airway pressure, may also be beneficial for management of COPD exacerbations in older people. A Cochrane review concluded that noninvasive positive airway pressure should be included as an adjunct therapy in suitable patients with respiratory failure from an episode of COPD exacerbation [73]. The challenge in an older population is identifying the suitable individual with respiratory failure for such therapy. Furthermore, 13-29% of patients are unable to tolerate the noninvasive mask.

Studies evaluating new anti-inflammatory drugs such as etanercept [74] and zileuton (anti-leukotriene inhibitor) [75], positive expiratory pressure therapy [76] and early inpatient respiratory rehabilitation [77] have not been found to be beneficial in terms of reducing hospital length of stay, readmission, treatment failure or recovery of physical function. A novel p38 mitogen activated protein kinase inhibitor, named BCT197 [78] and a highly selective β agonist, bedoradrine [65], are being evaluated for the management of acute exacerbations. Whether these agents have any additional benefits for older people will require further investigations.

END-OF-LIFE MANAGEMENT

Addressing advance directives in patients with end-stage COPD is an important aspect of care. In older people with end-stage COPD who choose not to have critical care treatment or withdraw from such treatment, palliative care is useful to relieve patients' symptoms. Opioids and benzodiazepines can be used to keep patients comfortable without markedly reducing time to death [79].

CONCLUSION

COPD affects as many as 14% of older adults and often has a progressive pattern that becomes more severe with advancing age. Spirometry assessment has an important place in diagnosis and staging of COPD, even in older age. As in other age groups, management of COPD should include smoking cessation, influenza and pneumococcal vaccinations, and the use of short- and long-acting bronchodilators. Selection of the appropriate inhaler device is important for older people with arthritis, poor manual dexterity, muscle weakness and visual or cognitive impairment. Other important treatment may include pulmonary rehabilitation, domiciliary oxygen therapy, noninvasive positive airway pressure and treatment of comorbidities. In older patients with end-stage COPD, palliative measures are important to relieve their symptoms.

CONFLICT OF INTEREST

The author confirms that author has no conflict of interest to declare for this publication.

ACKNOWLEDGEMENTS

Declared none.

KEY POINTS

- Chronic obstructive pulmonary disease (COPD) is common in the older population and is associated with significant disability.
- Spirometry which is useful for diagnosis and staging of COPD can be performed by most older people.
- Both nonpharmacological and pharmacological approaches need to be used to manage COPD in the elderly.
- Comorbidities are common in older people with COPD and should be managed accordingly.
- Palliative care and symptom management should be provided to patients with end-stage COPD.

REFERENCES

[1] Halbert RJ, Natoli JL, Gano A, Badamgarav E, Buist AS, Mannino DM. Global burden of COPD: systematic review and meta-analysis. Eur Respir J 2006; 28(3): 523-32. [http://dx.doi.org/10.1183/09031936.06.00124605] [PMID: 16611654]

[2] Mannino DM. COPD: epidemiology, prevalence, morbidity and mortality, and disease heterogeneity. Chest 2002; 121(5) (Suppl.): 121S-6S. [http://dx.doi.org/10.1378/chest.121.5_suppl.121S] [PMID: 12010839]

[3] Valente S, Pasciuto G, Bernabei R, Corbo GM. Do we need different treatments for very elderly COPD patients? Respiration 2010; 80(5): 357-68. [http://dx.doi.org/10.1159/000320221] [PMID: 20733280]

[4] Chan ED, Welsh CH. Geriatric respiratory medicine. Chest 1998; 114(6): 1704-33. [http://dx.doi.org/10.1378/chest.114.6.1704] [PMID: 9872208]

[5] Sharma G, Goodwin J. Effect of aging on respiratory system physiology and immunology. Clin Interv Aging 2006; 1(3): 253-60. [http://dx.doi.org/10.2147/ciia.2006.1.3.253] [PMID: 18046878]

[6] Rabe KF, Hurd S, Anzueto A, *et al.* Global strategy for the diagnosis, management, and prevention of chronic obstructive pulmonary disease: GOLD executive summary. Am J Respir Crit Care Med 2007; 176(6): 532-55. [http://dx.doi.org/10.1164/rccm.200703-456SO] [PMID: 17507545]

[7] Pezzoli L, Giardini G, Consonni S, *et al.* Quality of spirometric performance in older people. Age Ageing 2003; 32(1): 43-6. [http://dx.doi.org/10.1093/ageing/32.1.43] [PMID: 12540347]

[8] Hansen JE, Sun XG, Wasserman K. Spirometric criteria for airway obstruction: Use percentage of FEV1/FVC ratio below the fifth percentile, not < 70%. Chest 2007; 131(2): 349-55. [http://dx.doi.org/10.1378/chest.06-1349] [PMID: 17296632]

[9] Casanova C, Cote C, de Torres JP, *et al.* Inspiratory-to-total lung capacity ratio predicts mortality in patients with chronic obstructive pulmonary disease. Am J Respir Crit Care Med 2005; 171(6): 591-7. [http://dx.doi.org/10.1164/rccm.200407-867OC] [PMID: 15591470]

[10] Agustí A. Systemic effects of chronic obstructive pulmonary disease: what we know and what we don't know (but should). Proc Am Thorac Soc 2007; 4(7): 522-5. [http://dx.doi.org/10.1513/pats.200701-004FM] [PMID: 17878464]

[11] Yende S, Waterer GW, Tolley EA, *et al.* Inflammatory markers are associated with ventilatory limitation and muscle dysfunction in obstructive lung disease in well functioning elderly subjects. Thorax 2006; 61(1): 10-6. [http://dx.doi.org/10.1136/thx.2004.034181] [PMID: 16284220]

[12] Curkendall SM, DeLuise C, Jones JK, *et al.* Cardiovascular disease in patients with chronic obstructive pulmonary disease, Saskatchewan Canada cardiovascular disease in COPD patients. Ann Epidemiol 2006; 16(1): 63-70. [http://dx.doi.org/10.1016/j.annepidem.2005.04.008] [PMID: 16039877]

[13] de Lucas-Ramos P, Izquierdo-Alonso JL, Rodriguez-Gonzalez Moro JM, Frances JF, Lozano PV, Bellón-Cano JM. Chronic obstructive pulmonary disease as a cardiovascular risk factor. Results of a case-control study (CONSISTE study). Int J Chron Obstruct Pulmon Dis 2012; 7: 679-86. [PMID: 23055717]

[14] Samuels LE, Kaufman MS, Morris RJ, Promisloff R, Brockman SK. Coronary artery bypass grafting in patients with COPD. Chest 1998; 113(4): 878-82. [http://dx.doi.org/10.1378/chest.113.4.878] [PMID: 9554619]

[15] Sirak TE, Jelic S, Le Jemtel TH. Therapeutic update: non-selective beta- and alpha-adrenergic blockade in patients with coexistent chronic obstructive pulmonary disease and chronic heart failure. J Am Coll Cardiol 2004; 44(3): 497-502. [http://dx.doi.org/10.1016/j.jacc.2004.03.063] [PMID: 15358010]

[16] Divo M, Cote C, de Torres JP, *et al.* Comorbidities and risk of mortality in patients with chronic obstructive pulmonary disease. Am J Respir Crit Care Med 2012; 186(2): 155-61. [http://dx.doi.org/10.1164/rccm.201201-0034OC] [PMID: 22561964]

[17] Graat-Verboom L, Spruit MA, van den Borne BE, *et al.* Correlates of osteoporosis in chronic obstructive pulmonary disease: An underestimated systemic component. Respir Med 2009; 103(8): 1143-51. [http://dx.doi.org/10.1016/j.rmed.2009.02.014] [PMID: 19304474]

[18] Sin DD, Anthonisen NR, Soriano JB, Agusti AG. Mortality in COPD: Role of comorbidities. Eur Respir J 2006; 28(6): 1245-57. [http://dx.doi.org/10.1183/09031936.00133805] [PMID: 17138679]

[19] Miller J, Edwards LD, Agustí A, *et al.* Comorbidity, systemic inflammation and outcomes in the ECLIPSE cohort. Respir Med 2013; 107(9): 1376-84. [http://dx.doi.org/10.1016/j.rmed.2013.05.001] [PMID: 23791463]

[20] Harrison RA, Siminoski K, Vethanayagam D, Majumdar SR. Osteoporosis-related kyphosis and impairments in pulmonary function: a systematic review. J Bone Miner Res 2007; 22(3): 447-57.

[http://dx.doi.org/10.1359/jbmr.061202] [PMID: 17181402]

[21] Jones SE, Maddocks M, Kon SS, *et al.* Sarcopenia in COPD: prevalence, clinical correlates and response to pulmonary rehabilitation. Thorax 2015; 70(3): 213-8.
[http://dx.doi.org/10.1136/thoraxjnl-2014-206440] [PMID: 25561517]

[22] Anecchino C, Rossi E, Fanizza C, De Rosa M, Tognoni G, Romero M. Prevalence of chronic obstructive pulmonary disease and pattern of comorbidities in a general population. Int J Chron Obstruct Pulmon Dis 2007; 2(4): 567-74.
[PMID: 18268930]

[23] Schane RE, Walter LC, Dinno A, Covinsky KE, Woodruff PG. Prevalence and risk factors for depressive symptoms in persons with chronic obstructive pulmonary disease. J Gen Intern Med 2008; 23(11): 1757-62.
[http://dx.doi.org/10.1007/s11606-008-0749-z] [PMID: 18690488]

[24] Willgoss TG, Yohannes AM. Anxiety disorders in patients with COPD: a systematic review. Respir Care 2013; 58(5): 858-66.
[PMID: 22906542]

[25] Yohannes AM, Baldwin RC, Connolly MJ. Depression and anxiety in elderly outpatients with chronic obstructive pulmonary disease: prevalence, and validation of the BASDEC screening questionnaire. Int J Geriatr Psychiatry 2000; 15(12): 1090-6.
[http://dx.doi.org/10.1002/1099-1166(200012)15:12<1090::AID-GPS249>3.0.CO;2-L] [PMID: 11180464]

[26] Atlantis E, Fahey P, Cochrane B, Smith S. Bidirectional associations between clinically relevant depression or anxiety and COPD: a systematic review and meta-analysis. Chest 2013; 144(3): 766-77.
[http://dx.doi.org/10.1378/chest.12-1911] [PMID: 23429910]

[27] Wedzicha JA, Decramer M, Ficker JH, *et al.* Analysis of chronic obstructive pulmonary disease exacerbations with the dual bronchodilator QVA149 compared with glycopyrronium and tiotropium (SPARK): a randomised, double-blind, parallel-group study. Lancet Respir Med 2013; 1(3): 199-209.
[http://dx.doi.org/10.1016/S2213-2600(13)70052-3] [PMID: 24429126]

[28] Cafarella PA, Effing TW, Usmani ZA, Frith PA. Treatments for anxiety and depression in patients with chronic obstructive pulmonary disease: a literature review. Respirology 2012; 17(4): 627-38.
[http://dx.doi.org/10.1111/j.1440-1843.2012.02148.x] [PMID: 22309179]

[29] McKenzie DK, Frith PA, Burdon JG, Town GI. The COPDX Plan: Australian and New Zealand Guidelines for the management of Chronic Obstructive Pulmonary Disease 2003. Med J Aust 2003; 178 (Suppl.): S7-S39.
[PMID: 12633498]

[30] Abramson MJ, Crockett AJ, Frith PA, McDonald CF. COPDX: an update of guidelines for the management of chronic obstructive pulmonary disease with a review of recent evidence. Med J Aust 2006; 184(7): 342-5.
[PMID: 16584369]

[31] Celli BR. Update on the management of COPD. Chest 2008; 133(6): 1451-62.
[http://dx.doi.org/10.1378/chest.07-2061] [PMID: 18574288]

[32] Gupta P, O'Mahony MS. Potential adverse effects of bronchodilators in the treatment of airways obstruction in older people: recommendations for prescribing. Drugs Aging 2008; 25(5): 415-43. [http://dx.doi.org/10.2165/00002512-200825050-00005] [PMID: 18447405]

[33] Strassmann R, Bausch B, Spaar A, Kleijnen J, Braendli O, Puhan MA. Smoking cessation interventions in COPD: a network meta-analysis of randomised trials. Eur Respir J 2009; 34(3): 634-40. [http://dx.doi.org/10.1183/09031936.00167708] [PMID: 19357145]

[34] Tashkin DP, Rennard S, Hays JT, Ma W, Lawrence D, Lee TC. Effects of varenicline on smoking cessation in patients with mild to moderate COPD: a randomized controlled trial. Chest 2011; 139(3): 591-9. [http://dx.doi.org/10.1378/chest.10-0865] [PMID: 20864613]

[35] Garcia-Aymerich J, Lange P, Benet M, Schnohr P, Antó JM. Regular physical activity reduces hospital admission and mortality in chronic obstructive pulmonary disease: a population based cohort study. Thorax 2006; 61(9): 772-8. [http://dx.doi.org/10.1136/thx.2006.060145] [PMID: 16738033]

[36] Nazir SA, Al-Hamed MM, Erbland ML. Chronic obstructive pulmonary disease in the older patient. Clin Chest Med 2007; 28(4): 703-715, vi. [http://dx.doi.org/10.1016/j.ccm.2007.07.003] [PMID: 17967289]

[37] Ries AL, Bauldoff GS, Carlin BW, *et al.* Pulmonary rehabilitation: Joint ACCP/AACVPR evidence-based clinical practice guidelines. Chest 2007; 131(5) (Suppl.): 4S-42S. [http://dx.doi.org/10.1378/chest.06-2418] [PMID: 17494825]

[38] Vincken W. Bronchodilator treatment of stable COPD: long-acting anticholinergics. Eur Respir Rev 2005; 14: 23-31. [http://dx.doi.org/10.1183/09058180.05.00009403]

[39] Au DH, Udris EM, Fan VS, Curtis JR, McDonell MB, Fihn SD. Risk of mortality and heart failure exacerbations associated with inhaled beta-adrenoceptor agonists among patients with known left ventricular systolic dysfunction. Chest 2003; 123(6): 1964-9. [http://dx.doi.org/10.1378/chest.123.6.1964] [PMID: 12796175]

[40] Calverley PM, Anderson JA, Celli B, *et al.* Salmeterol and fluticasone propionate and survival in chronic obstructive pulmonary disease. N Engl J Med 2007; 356(8): 775-89. [http://dx.doi.org/10.1056/NEJMoa063070] [PMID: 17314337]

[41] Lee TA, Pickard AS, Au DH, Bartle B, Weiss KB. Risk for death associated with medications for recently diagnosed chronic obstructive pulmonary disease. Ann Intern Med 2008; 149(6): 380-90. [http://dx.doi.org/10.7326/0003-4819-149-6-200809160-00004] [PMID: 18794557]

[42] O'Donnell DE, Lam M, Webb KA. Spirometric correlates of improvement in exercise performance after anticholinergic therapy in chronic obstructive pulmonary disease. Am J Respir Crit Care Med 1999; 160(2): 542-9. [http://dx.doi.org/10.1164/ajrccm.160.2.9901038] [PMID: 10430726]

[43] Tashkin DP, Celli B, Senn S, *et al.* A 4-year trial of tiotropium in chronic obstructive pulmonary disease. N Engl J Med 2008; 359(15): 1543-54.

[http://dx.doi.org/10.1056/NEJMoa0805800] [PMID: 18836213]

[44] Kerwin E, Hébert J, Gallagher N, *et al.* Efficacy and safety of NVA237 *versus* placebo and tiotropium in patients with COPD: the GLOW2 study. Eur Respir J 2012; 40(5): 1106-14. [http://dx.doi.org/10.1183/09031936.00040712] [PMID: 23060624]

[45] D'Urzo A, Ferguson GT, van Noord JA, *et al.* Efficacy and safety of once-daily NVA237 in patients with moderate-to-severe COPD: the GLOW1 trial. Respir Res 2011; 12: 156. [http://dx.doi.org/10.1186/1465-9921-12-156] [PMID: 22151296]

[46] Ramsdell JW, Henderson S, Renvall MJ, Salmon DP, Ferguson P. Effects of theophylline and ipratropium on cognition in elderly patients with chronic obstructive pulmonary disease. Ann Allergy Asthma Immunol 1996; 76(4): 335-40. [http://dx.doi.org/10.1016/S1081-1206(10)60034-8] [PMID: 8612115]

[47] Singh S, Loke YK, Furberg CD. Inhaled anticholinergics and risk of major adverse cardiovascular events in patients with chronic obstructive pulmonary disease: a systematic review and meta-analysis. JAMA 2008; 300(12): 1439-50. [http://dx.doi.org/10.1001/jama.300.12.1439] [PMID: 18812535]

[48] Burge PS, Calverley PM, Jones PW, Spencer S, Anderson JA, Maslen TK. Randomised, double blind, placebo controlled study of fluticasone propionate in patients with moderate to severe chronic obstructive pulmonary disease: the ISOLDE trial. BMJ 2000; 320(7245): 1297-303. [http://dx.doi.org/10.1136/bmj.320.7245.1297] [PMID: 10807619]

[49] Suissa S, Barnes PJ. Inhaled corticosteroids in COPD: the case against. Eur Respir J 2009; 34(1): 13-6. [http://dx.doi.org/10.1183/09031936.00190908] [PMID: 19567599]

[50] Ernst P, Suissa S. Systemic effects of inhaled corticosteroids. Curr Opin Pulm Med 2012; 18(1): 85-9. [http://dx.doi.org/10.1097/MCP.0b013e32834dc51a] [PMID: 22112998]

[51] Aaron SD, Vandemheen KL, Fergusson D, *et al.* Tiotropium in combination with placebo, salmeterol, or fluticasone-salmeterol for treatment of chronic obstructive pulmonary disease: a randomized trial. Ann Intern Med 2007; 146(8): 545-55. [http://dx.doi.org/10.7326/0003-4819-146-8-200704170-00152] [PMID: 17310045]

[52] van Noord JA, Aumann JL, Janssens E, *et al.* Effects of tiotropium with and without formoterol on airflow obstruction and resting hyperinflation in patients with COPD. Chest 2006; 129(3): 509-17. [http://dx.doi.org/10.1378/chest.129.3.509] [PMID: 16537846]

[53] Connolly MJ. Inhaler technique of elderly patients: comparison of metered-dose inhalers and large volume spacer devices. Age Ageing 1995; 24(3): 190-2. [http://dx.doi.org/10.1093/ageing/24.3.190] [PMID: 7645436]

[54] Gooneratne NS, Patel NP, Corcoran A. Chronic obstructive pulmonary disease diagnosis and management in older adults. J Am Geriatr Soc 2010; 58(6): 1153-62. [http://dx.doi.org/10.1111/j.1532-5415.2010.02875.x] [PMID: 20936735]

[55] Jarvis S, Ind PW, Shiner RJ. Inhaled therapy in elderly COPD patients; time for re-evaluation? Age Ageing 2007; 36(2): 213-8. [http://dx.doi.org/10.1093/ageing/afl174] [PMID: 17267450]

[56] Dolovich MB, Ahrens RC, Hess DR, *et al.* Device selection and outcomes of aerosol therapy:

Evidence-based guidelines: American College of Chest Physicians/American College of Asthma, Allergy, and Immunology. Chest 2005; 127(1): 335-71.
[http://dx.doi.org/10.1378/chest.127.1.335] [PMID: 15654001]

[57] Allen S, Zamans S. A comparison of the turbohaler with a standard metered dose inhaler in elderly subjects with normal and impaired cognitive function. J HK Geriatr Soc 2000; 10: 75-7.

[58] Hak E, van Essen GA, Buskens E, Stalman W, de Melker RA. Is immunising all patients with chronic lung disease in the community against influenza cost effective? Evidence from a general practice based clinical prospective cohort study in Utrecht, The Netherlands. J Epidemiol Community Health 1998; 52(2): 120-5.
[http://dx.doi.org/10.1136/jech.52.2.120] [PMID: 9578860]

[59] Nichol KL, Margolis KL, Wuorenma J, Von Sternberg T. The efficacy and cost effectiveness of vaccination against influenza among elderly persons living in the community. N Engl J Med 1994; 331(12): 778-84.
[http://dx.doi.org/10.1056/NEJM199409223311206] [PMID: 8065407]

[60] Lederer DJ, Arcasoy SM. Update in surgical therapy for chronic obstructive pulmonary disease. Clin Chest Med 2007; 28(3): 639-653, vii. [vii.].
[http://dx.doi.org/10.1016/j.ccm.2007.05.004] [PMID: 17720050]

[61] Fishman A, Martinez F, Naunheim K, *et al.* A randomized trial comparing lung-volume-reduction surgery with medical therapy for severe emphysema. N Engl J Med 2003; 348(21): 2059-73.
[http://dx.doi.org/10.1056/NEJMoa030287] [PMID: 12759479]

[62] Long term domiciliary oxygen therapy in chronic hypoxic cor pulmonale complicating chronic bronchitis and emphysema. Report of the Medical Research Council Working Party. Lancet 1981; 1(8222): 681-6.
[PMID: 6110912]

[63] Nonoyama ML, Brooks D, Guyatt GH, Goldstein RS. Effect of oxygen on health quality of life in patients with chronic obstructive pulmonary disease with transient exertional hypoxemia. Am J Respir Crit Care Med 2007; 176(4): 343-9.
[http://dx.doi.org/10.1164/rccm.200702-308OC] [PMID: 17446339]

[64] Franciosi LG, Diamant Z, Banner KH, *et al.* Efficacy and safety of RPL554, a dual PDE3 and PDE4 inhibitor, in healthy volunteers and in patients with asthma or chronic obstructive pulmonary disease: findings from four clinical trials. Lancet Respir Med 2013; 1(9): 714-27.
[http://dx.doi.org/10.1016/S2213-2600(13)70187-5] [PMID: 24429275]

[65] Gross NJ. The COPD pipeline XXIV. COPD 2013; 10(5): 625-7.
[http://dx.doi.org/10.3109/15412555.2013.832093] [PMID: 24040908]

[66] Seemungal TA, Donaldson GC, Paul EA, Bestall JC, Jeffries DJ, Wedzicha JA. Effect of exacerbation on quality of life in patients with chronic obstructive pulmonary disease. Am J Respir Crit Care Med 1998; 157(5 Pt 1): 1418-22.
[http://dx.doi.org/10.1164/ajrccm.157.5.9709032] [PMID: 9603117]

[67] Kanner RE, Anthonisen NR, Connett JE. Lower respiratory illnesses promote FEV(1) decline in current smokers but not ex-smokers with mild chronic obstructive pulmonary disease: results from the lung health study. Am J Respir Crit Care Med 2001; 164(3): 358-64.

[http://dx.doi.org/10.1164/ajrccm.164.3.2010017] [PMID: 11500333]

[68] El Moussaoui R, Roede BM, Speelman P, Bresser P, Prins JM, Bossuyt PM. Short-course antibiotic treatment in acute exacerbations of chronic bronchitis and COPD: a meta-analysis of double-blind studies. Thorax 2008; 63(5): 415-22.
[http://dx.doi.org/10.1136/thx.2007.090613] [PMID: 18234905]

[69] Austin MA, Wills KE, Blizzard L, Walters EH, Wood-Baker R. Effect of high flow oxygen on mortality in chronic obstructive pulmonary disease patients in prehospital setting: randomised controlled trial. BMJ 2010; 341: c5462.
[http://dx.doi.org/10.1136/bmj.c5462] [PMID: 20959284]

[70] Ram FS, Rodriguez-Roisin R, Granados-Navarrete A, Garcia-Aymerich J, Barnes NC. Antibiotics for exacerbations of chronic obstructive pulmonary disease. Cochrane Database Syst Rev 2006; (2): CD004403.
[PMID: 16625602]

[71] Niewoehner DE, Erbland ML, Deupree RH, *et al.* Effect of systemic glucocorticoids on exacerbations of chronic obstructive pulmonary disease. N Engl J Med 1999; 340(25): 1941-7.
[http://dx.doi.org/10.1056/NEJM199906243402502] [PMID: 10379017]

[72] Aaron SD, Vandemheen KL, Hebert P, *et al.* Outpatient oral prednisone after emergency treatment of chronic obstructive pulmonary disease. N Engl J Med 2003; 348(26): 2618-25.
[http://dx.doi.org/10.1056/NEJMoa023161] [PMID: 12826636]

[73] Ram FS, Picot J, Lightowler J, Wedzicha JA. Non-invasive positive pressure ventilation for treatment of respiratory failure due to exacerbations of chronic obstructive pulmonary disease. Cochrane Database Syst Rev 2004; CD004104.

[74] Aaron SD, Vandemheen KL, Maltais F, *et al.* TNFα antagonists for acute exacerbations of COPD: a randomised double-blind controlled trial. Thorax 2013; 68(2): 142-8.
[http://dx.doi.org/10.1136/thoraxjnl-2012-202432] [PMID: 23161645]

[75] Woodruff PG, Albert RK, Bailey WC, *et al.* Randomized trial of zileuton for treatment of COPD exacerbations requiring hospitalization. COPD 2011; 8(1): 21-9.
[http://dx.doi.org/10.3109/15412555.2010.540273] [PMID: 21299475]

[76] Osadnik CR, McDonald CF, Miller BR, *et al.* The effect of positive expiratory pressure (PEP) therapy on symptoms, quality of life and incidence of re-exacerbation in patients with acute exacerbations of chronic obstructive pulmonary disease: a multicentre, randomised controlled trial. Thorax 2014; 69(2): 137-43.
[http://dx.doi.org/10.1136/thoraxjnl-2013-203425] [PMID: 24005444]

[77] Greening NJ, Williams JE, Hussain SF, *et al.* An early rehabilitation intervention to enhance recovery during hospital admission for an exacerbation of chronic respiratory disease: randomised controlled trial. BMJ 2014; 349: g4315.
[http://dx.doi.org/10.1136/bmj.g4315] [PMID: 25004917]

[78] Compton C, McBryan D, Bucchioni E, Patalano F. The Novartis view on emerging drugs and novel targets for the treatment of chronic obstructive pulmonary disease. Pulm Pharmacol Ther 2013; 26(5): 562-73.
[http://dx.doi.org/10.1016/j.pupt.2013.05.009] [PMID: 23748050]

[79] Shanawani H, Wenrich MD, Tonelli MR, Curtis JR. Meeting physicians' responsibilities in providing end-of-life care. Chest 2008; 133(3): 775-86.
[http://dx.doi.org/10.1378/chest.07-2177] [PMID: 18321905]

CHAPTER 8

Cancer in Older Adults: To Treat or Not to Treat?

Tuck Yean Yong[1,*], Kareeann Sok Fun Khow[2]

[1] *Internal Medicine, Flinders Private Hospital, Flinders Drive, Bedford Park, South Australia 5042, Australia*

[2] *Aged and Extended Care Services, The Queen Elizabeth Hospital and Department of Medicine, University of Adelaide, Adelaide, South Australia, Australia*

Abstract: The incidence of cancer in older people (aged ≥65 years) is about 8-fold higher than in the younger population and there is a growing number of cancer survivors living beyond the age of 65 years. When cancer is suspected or diagnosed in an older person, clinicians face many challenges related to diagnosis and management. Treatment decisions in older cancer patients need to take into account the individual's level of function and reserve. The best approach to assess an older individual's medical, psychological and functional capabilities is through the application of a Comprehensive Geriatric Assessment (CGA). CGA has been shown to predict treatment outcomes and survival in oncology settings as well as guide the implementation of multidisciplinary interventions. The goals of cancer treatment in older adults should be cure if possible and prolongation of active life expectancy as well as maintaining quality of life. There is still a dearth of clinical trials evaluating cancer treatment in the older people; an issue which needs to be addressed urgently as the population ages.

Keywords: Cancer, Chemotherapy, Diagnosis, Frailty, Geriatric, Malignancy, Multidisciplinary, Older, Oncology, Quality of life, Survivorship, Treatment.

INTRODUCTION

The incidence of many cancers increases with age [1]. As a result of population ageing, cancers are increasingly diagnosed. In many countries, more than 50% of

* **Correspondence author Tuck Yean Yong:** Internal Medicine, Flinders Private Hospital, Flinders Drive, Bedford Park, South Australia 5042, Australia; Tel: +61 8 8241 2121; Fax: +61 8 8240 0879; E-mail: tyyong@hotmail.com.

newly diagnosed cancers occur among people aged ≥65 years [2].

Cancer is a major cause of mortality worldwide, accounting for an estimated 9.9 million yearly, of which 54% occur in people aged ≥60 years [1]. As early detection and treatment options have expanded, long-term cancer survival has improved and the number of survivors living in their older age is growing [3].

Cancer care in the older people is complex and challenging. When cancer is suspected or diagnosed in older people, multiple challenges arise including diagnostic and treatment uncertainties because of limited evidence on risk-benefit [4]. In addition, providing comprehensive survivorship care to older people can be challenging.

The purpose of this chapter is to review the clinical differences in older cancer patients, approach to their management, provision of survivorship care and gaps in evidence related to their care.

CANCER IN DIFFERENT AGE GROUPS

In contrast to younger people, the presentations of cancers among elderly are often non-specific and may be obscured by other co-existing conditions which can lead to underdiagnosis and diagnosis at a more advanced stage [5]. In older people, multiple malignancies are common at presentation, occurring in up to 20% [6]. Another difference for older people with cancer is the higher frequency of functional disability; 20% have impaired activities of daily living (ADL) and 70% have impaired instrumental activities of daily living (IADL) [7, 8]. The state of increased frailty reduces the benefits of cancer treatment and increases their vulnerability to therapy-related complications [9].

Ageing is characterised by decreased homeostatic reserve which can affect cardiovascular, renal, immunological and haematological systems which are relevant to cancer treatment [10]. In addition, age-related changes in drug pharmacokinetics, pharmacodynamics and metabolism need to be taken into account in treating older people with cancer. Other important differences to take into consideration include polypharmacy, social isolation and more competing concurrent diseases which are more common in the older adults [11, 12]. Geriatric syndromes such as cognitive impairment, delirium, malnutrition and falls can affect cancer therapy or arise as complications of treatment [13].

The older population is heterogenous and functional reserve of organ systems are poorly reflected by chronological age. As a result there is great variability in health and functional status among older adults of the same chronological age. In contrast, physiological age is more important in decision-making for cancer treatment.

ASSESSMENT OF OLDER PEOPLE WITH CANCER

Comprehensive geriatric assessment (CGA) is one of the most useful ways of estimating one's physiological age in cancer care (Table **1**). CGA is a multidimensional process focused on evaluating an older person's medical, psychological and functional status to facilitate integrated planning of treatment [14]. In a meta-analysis of 28 controlled trials, the use of CGA was associated with reduced risk of mortality, reduced hospital readmissions, improved physical function and increased likelihood of living at home [15]. In oncology clinical trials, CGA was useful in identifying unsuspected geriatric problems and syndromes [16 - 18], predicting treatment outcome and survival [19 - 22] and developing multidisciplinary interventions [23, 24].

Table 1. Comprehensive Geriatric Assessment domains and potential clinical applications.

Domain	Clinical Application
Functional status Activities of daily living Instrumental activities of daily living	Estimate life expectancy Determine functional independence
Comorbidity Comorbidity indices	Estimate life expectancy
Cognition Mini-mental State Examination	Determine life expectancy and functional independence
Mood Geriatric Depression Scale	Indicate motivation to engage in treatment
Nutrition Mini Nutritional Assessment	Potentially reversible condition
Polypharmacy	Risk of drug interactions

(Table 1) contd.....

Domain	Clinical Application
Geriatric syndromes Delirium Falls and fractures Incontinence	Estimate life expectancy Determine functional independence Identify potentially reversible syndrome(s)

CGA in older people with cancers can reveal unsuspected geriatric syndromes including dementia, delirium, depression, weight loss, malnutrition and functional disability; changing cancer treatments in 21-49% of those assessed [16 - 18]. Identification of delirium in older patients with cancers is important because potentially reversible causes can be treated [25].

In older cancer patients, CGA can predict treatment outcomes and complications of surgery and chemotherapy. Dependence in IADL can predict a poorer surgical outcome [19]. In one study of older people assessed for chemotherapy, a score including hearing loss, fall within 6 months, IADL (ability to take medications), difficulty to walk one block and reduced social activity, predicted chemotherapy toxicity; while the Karnofsky performance status did not [20]. In older people with diffuse large-cell lymphoma, the CGA was more effective than clinical judgement in identifying those who can benefit from aggressive immunochemotherapy [21].

TREATMENT CONSIDERATIONS FOR OLDER PEOPLE WITH CANCER

Management decisions of older people with cancer have to be guided by many considerations that may include the functional level, tolerance to and benefit-t--risk ratio of diagnostic and therapeutic interventions, socio-economic support, life expectancy and patients' values and wishes. Generally, the goals of treatment in the older population with cancer are cure if possible, prolongation of survival (possibly free of significant disability), symptom alleviation and enhancement of the quality of life. In older people, preservation of function and active life expectancy are important goals [4]. Active life expectancy is described as a period of time during which a person remains functionally independent, which is important in maintaining quality of life.

The benefit of systemic cancer treatment may decrease with age while risks may increase because of reduced life expectancy and tolerance of stress [26]. Even in the most fit of older people, age is a risk factor for some complications of chemotherapy such as myelosuppression, mucositis, peripheral neuropathy and cardiomyopathy [26].

Ageism can be a barrier to the reception of adequate cancer treatment. In one study, the main obstacle to clinical trial participation of older women with breast cancer was the reluctance of physicians to offer experimental treatment to this group [27]. In contrast, in a study of nearly 1500 older people (age ≥70 years) with chronic lymphocytic leukaemia not eligible for more aggressive treatment (such as combination of fludarabine, cyclophosphamide and rituximab) were randomized to receive chlorambucil or chlorambucil plus rituximab or obinutuzumab [28]. The study showed that disease-free and overall survival rates were better in patients treated with obinutuzumab.

CANCER SURVIVORSHIP IN OLDER ADULTS

As early detection and treatment options for cancer have grown, long-term survival has improved and increasing number of survivors is living into older age (>65 years) [29]. Providing comprehensive survivorship care to older people can be challenging because they usually receive care in the community, rarely included in clinical trials and often present with competing illnesses that limit therapeutic options. Long-term survivorship care requires periodic monitoring for cancer recurrence, new cancers, late effects and long-term symptoms from treatment, health promotion and meeting psychosocial needs [30]. Both cancer specialists and primary care physicians are involved in the long-term follow-up.

Three survival care models have been proposed: (a) Oncologist-led care, (b) Community-based shared care, and (c) Team-based survivorship clinic. There is still disagreement about the preferred model [31]. Regardless of the model used, care of older cancer survivors must address the need for good inter-disciplinary communication especially on comanagement of common chronic conditions such as heart disease, diabetes mellitus and arthritis. Older cancer patients have more comorbidities than non-cancer patients, and studies have identified that some may receive lower quality of care [32, 33]. The use of CGA prior to initiating cancer treatment can be useful in informing survivorship care of older patients [34].

MODELS OF CARE

Collaboration between geriatrician and cancer specialists should become the cornerstone of integrating principles of geriatric care into oncological management of older people with cancer. A structured Geriatric Oncology Program that brings together cancer specialists, geriatricians, nurses, physiotherapists and social workers should be implemented more widely [35, 36]. This approach is consistent with the recommendation of the International Society of Geriatric Oncology that every older adult with cancer should have an assessment to identify those who are frail [37]. Instead of excluding frail older people from standard cancer treatment, some of them may still benefit from an individualised intervention based on CGA to manage issues that might limit oncological therapy [5, 37]. The important areas of CGA to focus in an older cancer patient include functional status, comorbidity and its severity, medication use and potential drug-drug interactions, nutritional status, cognition and social support. Studies of Geriatric Oncology Programmes and Onco-Geriatric approaches have shown promising outcomes in improving selection of older people for appropriate intervention [19, 38].

CHALLENGES IN CANCER CARE OF OLDER PEOPLE

Data relating to cancer treatment in the older population are limited because this group of patients are often under-represented in clinical trials [39]. Age should not be the sole criterion for excluding an older person with cancer from a clinical trial. Phase 2 trials including older people are necessary to establish the pharmacology of new agents in this group of patients. Phase 3 trials that study the older population should stratify these participants according to treatment risks and life expectancy.

CONCLUSION

Increasing age is associated with increasing functional decline, comorbidity and declining physiological reserve. As a result older people with cancers are at increased risk of treatment-related adverse effects, drug interactions and onset of geriatric syndromes, compared to their peers without cancer. The management of older people with cancer will benefit from the use of CGA and the contribution from a geriatrician. Treatment should be personalized and take into consideration an older individual's medical, psychological and functional status.

CONFLICT OF INTEREST

The author confirms that author has no conflict of interest to declare for this publication.

ACKNOWLEDGEMENTS

Declared none.

KEY POINTS

- The incidence of cancer is higher in the older age (>65 years) group.
- Frailty in older people may reduce the benefits of cancer treatment and increased vulnerability to complications related to therapies.
- Comprehensive Geriatric Assessment is a useful approach to evaluate older people with cancer to identify those who will potentially benefit from treatment.
- Care of older cancer survivors requires knowledge of geriatric medicine and care coordination among multiple health providers.
- More clinical trials are needed in the older population so that future treatment can be more evidence-based.

REFERENCES

[1] Torre LA, Bray F, Siegel RL, Ferlay J, Lortet-Tieulent J, Jemal A. Global cancer statistics, 2012. CA Cancer J Clin 2015; 65(2): 87-108.
[http://dx.doi.org/10.3322/caac.21262] [PMID: 25651787]

[2] Prince MJ, Wu F, Guo Y, *et al.* The burden of disease in older people and implications for health policy and practice. Lancet 2015; 385(9967): 549-62.
[http://dx.doi.org/10.1016/S0140-6736(14)61347-7] [PMID: 25468153]

[3] de Moor JS, Mariotto AB, Parry C, *et al.* Cancer survivors in the United States: prevalence across the survivorship trajectory and implications for care. Cancer Epidemiol Biomarkers Prev 2013; 22(4): 561-70.
[http://dx.doi.org/10.1158/1055-9965.EPI-12-1356] [PMID: 23535024]

[4] Balducci L, Aapro M. Complicated and complex: helping the older patient with cancer to exit the

labyrinth. J Geriatr Oncol 2014; 5(1): 116-8.
[http://dx.doi.org/10.1016/j.jgo.2013.11.003] [PMID: 24484725]

[5] Balducci L, Colloca G, Cesari M, Gambassi G. Assessment and treatment of elderly patients with cancer. Surg Oncol 2010; 19(3): 117-23.
[http://dx.doi.org/10.1016/j.suronc.2009.11.008] [PMID: 20006489]

[6] Luciani A, Balducci L. Multiple primary malignancies. Semin Oncol 2004; 31(2): 264-73.
[http://dx.doi.org/10.1053/j.seminoncol.2003.12.035] [PMID: 15112155]

[7] Extermann M, Overcash J, Lyman GH, Parr J, Balducci L. Comorbidity and functional status are independent in older cancer patients. J Clin Oncol 1998; 16(4): 1582-7.
[PMID: 9552069]

[8] Repetto L, Fratino L, Audisio RA, *et al.* Comprehensive geriatric assessment adds information to Eastern Cooperative Oncology Group performance status in elderly cancer patients: an Italian Group for Geriatric Oncology Study. J Clin Oncol 2002; 20(2): 494-502.
[http://dx.doi.org/10.1200/JCO.20.2.494] [PMID: 11786579]

[9] Balducci L. Frailty: a common pathway in aging and cancer. Interdiscip Top Gerontol 2013; 38: 61-72.
[http://dx.doi.org/10.1159/000343586] [PMID: 23503516]

[10] Cohen HJ. Biology of aging as related to cancer. Cancer 1994; 74(7) (Suppl.): 2092-100.
[http://dx.doi.org/10.1002/1097-0142(19941001)74:7+<2092::AID-CNCR2820741717>3.0.CO;2-G] [PMID: 8087776]

[11] McKenna RJ Sr. Clinical aspects of cancer in the elderly. Treatment decisions, treatment choices, and follow-up. Cancer 1994; 74(7) (Suppl.): 2107-17.
[http://dx.doi.org/10.1002/1097-0142(19941001)74:7+<2107::AID-CNCR2820741719>3.0.CO;2-1] [PMID: 8087778]

[12] Lees J, Chan A. Polypharmacy in elderly patients with cancer: clinical implications and management. Lancet Oncol 2011; 12(13): 1249-57.
[http://dx.doi.org/10.1016/S1470-2045(11)70040-7] [PMID: 21741307]

[13] Mohile SG, Fan L, Reeve E, *et al.* Association of cancer with geriatric syndromes in older Medicare beneficiaries. J Clin Oncol 2011; 29(11): 1458-64.
[http://dx.doi.org/10.1200/JCO.2010.31.6695] [PMID: 21402608]

[14] Extermann M. Comprehensive geriatric assessment basics for the cancer professional. J Oncol Manag 2003; 12(2): 13-7.
[PMID: 12699111]

[15] Stuck AE, Siu AL, Wieland GD, Adams J, Rubenstein LZ. Comprehensive geriatric assessment: a meta-analysis of controlled trials. Lancet 1993; 342(8878): 1032-6.
[http://dx.doi.org/10.1016/0140-6736(93)92884-V] [PMID: 8105269]

[16] Chaïbi P, Magné N, Breton S, *et al.* Influence of geriatric consultation with comprehensive geriatric assessment on final therapeutic decision in elderly cancer patients. Crit Rev Oncol Hematol 2011; 79(3): 302-7.
[http://dx.doi.org/10.1016/j.critrevonc.2010.08.004] [PMID: 20888781]

[17] Caillet P, Canoui-Poitrine F, Vouriot J, *et al.* Comprehensive geriatric assessment in the decision-making process in elderly patients with cancer: ELCAPA study. J Clin Oncol 2011; 29(27): 3636-42. [http://dx.doi.org/10.1200/JCO.2010.31.0664] [PMID: 21709194]

[18] Flood KL, Carroll MB, Le CV, Ball L, Esker DA, Carr DB. Geriatric syndromes in elderly patients admitted to an oncology-acute care for elders unit. J Clin Oncol 2006; 24(15): 2298-303. [http://dx.doi.org/10.1200/JCO.2005.02.8514] [PMID: 16710027]

[19] Pope D, Ramesh H, Gennari R, *et al.* Pre-operative assessment of cancer in the elderly (PACE): a comprehensive assessment of underlying characteristics of elderly cancer patients prior to elective surgery. Surg Oncol 2006; 15(4): 189-97. [http://dx.doi.org/10.1016/j.suronc.2007.04.009] [PMID: 17531743]

[20] Hurria A, Togawa K, Mohile SG, *et al.* Predicting chemotherapy toxicity in older adults with cancer: a prospective multicenter study. J Clin Oncol 2011; 29(25): 3457-65. [http://dx.doi.org/10.1200/JCO.2011.34.7625] [PMID: 21810685]

[21] Tucci A, Ferrari S, Bottelli C, Borlenghi E, Drera M, Rossi G. A comprehensive geriatric assessment is more effective than clinical judgment to identify elderly diffuse large cell lymphoma patients who benefit from aggressive therapy. Cancer 2009; 115(19): 4547-53. [http://dx.doi.org/10.1002/cncr.24490] [PMID: 19562776]

[22] Kanesvaran R, Li H, Koo KN, Poon D. Analysis of prognostic factors of comprehensive geriatric assessment and development of a clinical scoring system in elderly Asian patients with cancer. J Clin Oncol 2011; 29(27): 3620-7. [http://dx.doi.org/10.1200/JCO.2010.32.0796] [PMID: 21859998]

[23] Rao AV, Hsieh F, Feussner JR, Cohen HJ. Geriatric evaluation and management units in the care of the frail elderly cancer patient. J Gerontol A Biol Sci Med Sci 2005; 60(6): 798-803. [http://dx.doi.org/10.1093/gerona/60.6.798] [PMID: 15983186]

[24] Extermann M, Meyer J, McGinnis M, *et al.* A comprehensive geriatric intervention detects multiple problems in older breast cancer patients. Crit Rev Oncol Hematol 2004; 49(1): 69-75. [http://dx.doi.org/10.1016/S1040-8428(03)00099-4] [PMID: 14734156]

[25] Weinrich S, Sarna L. Delirium in the older person with cancer. Cancer 1994; 74(7) (Suppl.): 2079-91. [http://dx.doi.org/10.1002/1097-0142(19941001)74:7+<2079::AID-CNCR2820741716>3.0.CO;2-0] [PMID: 8087775]

[26] Hoffe S, Balducci L. Cancer and age: general considerations. Clin Geriatr Med 2012; 28(1): 1-18. [http://dx.doi.org/10.1016/j.cger.2011.09.001] [PMID: 22326032]

[27] Kemeny MM, Peterson BL, Kornblith AB, *et al.* Barriers to clinical trial participation by older women with breast cancer. J Clin Oncol 2003; 21(12): 2268-75. [http://dx.doi.org/10.1200/JCO.2003.09.124] [PMID: 12805325]

[28] Goede V, Fischer K, Busch R, *et al.* Obinutuzumab plus chlorambucil in patients with CLL and coexisting conditions. N Engl J Med 2014; 370(12): 1101-10. [http://dx.doi.org/10.1056/NEJMoa1313984] [PMID: 24401022]

[29] Siegel R, DeSantis C, Virgo K, *et al.* Cancer treatment and survivorship statistics, 2012. CA Cancer J Clin 2012; 62(4): 220-41.

[http://dx.doi.org/10.3322/caac.21149] [PMID: 22700443]

[30] Chubak J, Tuzzio L, Hsu C, *et al.* Providing care for cancer survivors in integrated health care delivery systems: practices, challenges, and research opportunities. J Oncol Pract 2012; 8(3): 184-9. [http://dx.doi.org/10.1200/JOP.2011.000312] [PMID: 22942814]

[31] Gage EA, Pailler M, Zevon MA, *et al.* Structuring survivorship care: discipline-specific clinician perspectives. J Cancer Surviv 2011; 5(3): 217-25. [http://dx.doi.org/10.1007/s11764-011-0174-x] [PMID: 21311997]

[32] Smith AW, Reeve BB, Bellizzi KM, *et al.* Cancer, comorbidities, and health-related quality of life of older adults. Health Care Financ Rev 2008; 29(4): 41-56. [PMID: 18773613]

[33] Snyder CF, Frick KD, Herbert RJ, *et al.* Quality of care for comorbid conditions during the transition to survivorship: differences between cancer survivors and noncancer controls. J Clin Oncol 2013; 31(9): 1140-8. [http://dx.doi.org/10.1200/JCO.2012.43.0272] [PMID: 23401438]

[34] Hamaker ME, Jonker JM, de Rooij SE, Vos AG, Smorenburg CH, van Munster BC. Frailty screening methods for predicting outcome of a comprehensive geriatric assessment in elderly patients with cancer: a systematic review. Lancet Oncol 2012; 13(10): e437-44. [http://dx.doi.org/10.1016/S1470-2045(12)70259-0] [PMID: 23026829]

[35] Monfardini S, Aapro MS, Bennett JM, *et al.* Organization of the clinical activity of geriatric oncology: report of a SIOG (International Society of Geriatric Oncology) task force. Crit Rev Oncol Hematol 2007; 62(1): 62-73. [http://dx.doi.org/10.1016/j.critrevonc.2006.10.003] [PMID: 17300950]

[36] Pallis AG, Fortpied C, Wedding U, *et al.* EORTC elderly task force position paper: approach to the older cancer patient. Eur J Cancer 2010; 46(9): 1502-13. [http://dx.doi.org/10.1016/j.ejca.2010.02.022] [PMID: 20227872]

[37] Extermann M, Aapro M, Bernabei R, *et al.* Use of comprehensive geriatric assessment in older cancer patients: recommendations from the task force on CGA of the International Society of Geriatric Oncology (SIOG). Crit Rev Oncol Hematol 2005; 55(3): 241-52. [http://dx.doi.org/10.1016/j.critrevonc.2005.06.003] [PMID: 16084735]

[38] Cesari M, Colloca G, Cerullo F, *et al.* Onco-geriatric approach for the management of older patients with cancer. J Am Med Dir Assoc 2011; 12(2): 153-9. [http://dx.doi.org/10.1016/j.jamda.2010.06.008] [PMID: 21266292]

[39] Hutchins LF, Unger JM, Crowley JJ, Coltman CA Jr, Albain KS. Underrepresentation of patients 65 years of age or older in cancer-treatment trials. N Engl J Med 1999; 341(27): 2061-7. [http://dx.doi.org/10.1056/NEJM199912303412706] [PMID: 10615079]

CHAPTER 9

Overcoming Osteoarthritis in Old Age

Kareeann Sok Fun Khow*

Aged and Extended Care Services, The Queen Elizabeth Hospital and Department of Medicine, University of Adelaide, Adelaide, South Australia, Australia

Abstract: Osteoarthritis is a common diagnosis in older people aged 65 years and above, which causes significant pain leading to disability and decreased quality of life. Nonpharmacological measures such as exercise and footwear are essential in the management of osteoarthritis-related pain and disability in the older population if medication adverse effects and polypharmacy are to be avoided. Pharmacological approaches to pain management should complement nonpharmacological treatment. Most drug therapies give mild-to-moderate pain relief but their long-term efficacy and safety in older people remain undetermined. In older patients with severe osteoarthritis of the hips or knees responding poorly to analgesics, total joint arthroplasty offers the most effective intervention for those who are fit for surgery.

Keywords: Analgesia, Arthroplasty, Elderly, Exercise, Footwear, Knee, Hip, Osteoarthritis, Pain management, Physical therapy, Surgery.

INTRODUCTION

Osteoarthritis is one of the leading chronic condition causing functional decline and morbidity in older people aged ≥65 years [1]. Osteoarthritis involving joints in the lower limbs is a leading cause of impaired mobility and disability in older people [2]. The prevalence of osteoarthritis increases with age and with an ageing population, this condition will have a significant burden on health care [3]. Management of osteoarthritis-related pain is a challenge in older people. In this age group, undertreatment of pain can lead to decreased mobility, cognition and

* **Correspondence author Kareeann Sok Fun Khow:** Aged and Extended Care Services, The Queen Elizabeth Hospital, Woodville Road, Woodville South, South Australia 5011, Australia; Tel: +61 8 8222 6000; Fax: +61 8 8222 8593; E-mail: kareeann.khow@adelaide.edu.au.

Tuck Yean Yong (Ed)

self-related health, which can threaten independence [4, 5]. Older people often have multiple chronic conditions that can compound osteoarthritis-related pain, a high rate of polypharmacy and increased susceptibility to the adverse effects of analgesics [6].

This chapter will review the nonpharmacological, pharmacological and surgical therapy for osteoarthritis of the knee and hip with specific reference to older people.

DIAGNOSIS AND CLINICAL FEATURES

The pain of osteoarthritis is usually activity-related. Patients with knee involvement may report that their legs "give way", which is known as instability symptom. With knee osteoarthritis, tenderness at the junction of the femur and tibia or an effusion may be present. Varus (bowlegged) or valgus (knock-kneed) deformity usually signifies marked malalignment which these changes are risk factors for worsening radiographic disease and functional limitations [7]. One of the useful signs for recognising osteoarthritis of the hip is pain that is aggravated by internal or external rotation of the hip while the knee is in full extension [8].

Blood tests are usually not indicated in the evaluation of chronic knee or hip pain unless clinical features are suggestive of rheumatoid arthritis or other forms of inflammatory arthritis. Radiological imaging is required in the workup if pain is nocturnal or not related to activities. In people with osteoarthritis, radiological findings do not correlate well with the severity of pain and radiographs of the affected joint may even appear normal in people with the condition [9].

NONPHARMACOLOGICAL INTERVENTIONS

Nonpharmacological measures have an important role in the management of osteoarthritis-related pain and disability in the older population if medication adverse effects and polypharmacy are to be avoided. The American College of Rheumatology (ACR) recommends that management of osteoarthritis should include measures such as self-management programs, social support, weight loss and appropriate footwear [10].

Both the ACR and the Osteoarthritis Arthritis Research Society International

(OARSI) recommend using lateral-wedged insoles for osteoarthritis [8, 11]. Lateral-wedged orthotics decreases the degree of varus misalignment at the knee [12]. Randomized controlled trials have shown that lateral wedged orthotics in knee osteoarthritis can decrease oral analgesic use at 6 months and 2 years but no improvement in pain or function was observed [13, 14]. However the long-term effects of this approach are currently unknown. Since an insole is a simple and inexpensive measure, lateral wedged orthotics are an option in ambulating older people with knee osteoarthritis who need to reduce non-steroidal anti-inflammatory drugs (NSAID) use.

A systematic review evaluating patellar taping in knee pain with varus malalignment found that pain was significantly reduced but only three studies included older people [15]. However further work is required to determine the efficacy of patellar taping in knee osteoarthritis.

Physical therapy to strengthen muscle function and aerobic exercises can improve osteoarthritis symptoms [16]. A systematic review of 12 randomized controlled trials (RCTs) showed that exercise therapy and manual joint mobilisation was superior to either strength training or exercise therapy alone in medial knee osteoarthritis, but all three modalities improved physical function and pain [17]. Physical therapy is even more important in older people with multiple comorbidities and requires rehabilitation.

Obesity has been considered the single most "modifiable" risk factor knee osteoarthritis [18, 19]. A meta-analysis has shown that weight loss of 5% within a 20-week period is associated with pain and functional improvement in knee osteoarthritis [20]. However the effectiveness of this approach in older people with osteoarthritis have not been examined in light of potential adverse outcomes associated with weight loss in this age group [21].

PHARMACOLOGICAL THERAPY

Oral Analgesics

NSAID is effective in treating pain as well as reducing joint swelling and stiffness in osteoarthritis and is considered the first-line treatment for mild to moderate pain [22]. A meta-analysis of 27 RCTs has confirmed the superiority of NSAID over paracetamol for relieving pain in knee osteoarthritis [23]. In a large RCT, selective cyclooxygenase-2 (COX-2) inhibitors reduce pain as effectively as non-selective NSAID [24]. However, non-selective NSAID was associated with higher gastrointestinal adverse effects including ulceration, bleeding and perforation [24]. In patients at risk of gastrointestinal adverse events, concomitant use of proton pump inhibitors is generally recommended. A meta-analysis found that combining a proton pump inhibitor with NSAID use reduced the relative risk of dyspepsia by 66% and the absolute risk by 9% compared with NSAID alone [25]. In addition to gastrointestinal and renal adverse effects, NSAID is also associated with increased cardiovascular complications which are a concern for the older population [26]. The optimum duration of NSAID is uncertain. A meta-analysis of RCTs found no clear association between the duration of taking selective or non-selective NSAID and the risk of cardiovascular events [27]. One study found continuous celecoxib use to be slightly more effective than intermittent use on pain and function, with comparable rates of discontinuation due to adverse events [28]. No studies have assessed harms from serious gastrointestinal and cardiovascular events associated with intermittent dosing of NSAID.

Paracetamol (acetaminophen) was once regarded as the general analgesic of choice for mild to moderate pain in osteoarthritis but it is no longer recommended as first line treatment by recent guidelines [29, 30]. A meta-analysis has reported little improvement in pain in the setting of osteoarthritis [31]. Furthermore a RCT found that paracetamol 4 g/day was not superior to placebo for pain management in knee osteoarthritis [32]. Besides its lack of efficacy in managing osteoarthritis, concerns about adverse effects with paracetamol have emerged when used in high doses and in patients with multiple comorbidities which can be common among older people. Increased risk of gastrointestinal events and multi-organ failure has been reported with supratherapeutic doses of paracetamol [33]. The Nurses' Health Study found that prolonged use of paracetamol (>22 days/month) was associated with an increased risk of cardiovascular events (relative risk 1.4; 95% confidence interval [CI] 1.1-1.6), similar to that of NSAID use [34]. Furthermore, one study of elderly subject reported that the risk of gastrointestinal-related hospitalizations was higher with the combination of paracetamol and NSAID (hazard ratio [HR] 2.55, 95% CI 1.98-3.28) compared with paracetamol alone (>3 g/day) (HR 1.20, 95% CI 1.03-1.40) and NSAID alone (HR 1.63, 95% CI 1.44-1.85) [35].

Tramadol is a weak atypical opioid analgesic. In a meta-analysis of eleven RCTs, tramadol reduced osteoarthritis-related pain but the effect was small [36]. In a post-hoc analysis of older participants in a RCT with tramadol have shown improvement in pain and sleep-related outcomes but adverse effects were moderately high including constipation (28%), nausea (23%) and pre-syncopal symptom (23%) [37]. Pre-syncopal symptom is a concern in older people because this can increase the risk of falls and related injuries.

Duloxetine is a serotonin and noradrenaline reuptake inhibitor and can be used to treat chronic musculoskeletal pain including osteoarthritis. The use of duloxetine is based on the premise that pain is multifactorial, with depression and neuropathic pain compounding the overall pain syndrome. In a placebo-controlled RCT, duloxetine (60-120 mg/day) produced significant improvement in pain control related to knee osteoarthritis and physical function after 13 weeks [38]. It can be a potential adjunct to conventional osteoarthritis treatment [39]. However, common adverse effects of duloxetine include nausea, constipation, fatigue, dry mouth and decreased appetite [39].

Opioids are usually used for osteoarthritis pain when other oral analgesics and non-drug interventions are ineffective [40]. In a systematic review of non-tramadol opioids including codeine, oxycodone, oxymorphone, morphine and transdermal fentanyl, these opioids had a small benefit in pain control and improving function over placebo but rates of serious adverse effects and dropouts were higher [40]. The usefulness of opioids in the long-term management of osteoarthritis is limited [41]. Although not specific for older people, opioids have an increased risk of adverse events compared with NSAID, including fractures (HR 4.47, 95% CI 3.12-6.41), cardiovascular events (HR 1.77 95% CI 1.39-2.24) and all-cause mortality (HR 1.87, 95% CI 1.39-2.53) [42]. Furthermore users were four times more likely to discontinue opioids compared with placebo, due to an adverse event (RR 4.05, 95% CI 3.06-5.38) [41].

Topical or Transdermal Agents

Topical capsaicin is recommended for management of pain in osteoarthritis [11]. It can be used as an alternative or an adjunct to standard drug treatment. A systematic review of RCTs found topical capsaicin to be superior to placebo for knee osteoarthritis and reduces pain by 50% [43]. In older patients, attention to application technique and skin integrity should be taken to avoid local irritation.

The use of topical NSAID for two to four weeks has been found to be efficacious in the management of knee osteoarthritis in two meta-analyses [44, 45]. The efficacy of topical NSAID in osteoarthritis is greater than placebo and comparable with oral NSAID [46]. This method of drug delivery reduces the gastrointestinal adverse effects seen with oral administration [47].

The safety of diclofenac sodium 1% gel has been shown in the older population in a 12-month post-hoc analysis of patients with knee osteoarthritis [48]. In this study, the overall rates of cardiovascular and gastrointestinal adverse events were similar for people under and over 65 years of age [48] . However, one of the adverse effects of topical NSAID is local irritation, which can occur in about 4% of users [47]. To date, most studies of topical NSAID have focused on individuals with knee osteoarthritis so the benefits in people with multiple joint osteoarthritis remain uncertain.

Although no RCT has tested the efficacy of 5% lidocaine transdermal patches in osteoarthritis, two open-label trials have reported reduction in knee pain after two weeks [49, 50]. Adverse effects are minimal with transdermal lidocaine except for local skin irritation. However dizziness can occur with overdosage and patients or caregivers must be advised to apply patches only for 12 continuous hours within a 24 h period.

Intraarticular Agents

Intraarticular corticosteroid (IAC) injections have been used to treat knee and hip osteoarthritis [10, 11]. A Cochrane review of 28 RCTs on IAC in knee osteoarthritis found that there was a significant reduction in pain one week post injection which was maximal at 2-3 weeks after administration [51]. No significant benefit has been observed beyond 3 weeks but long-term effects have only been investigated by a few small studies. However, no functional improvement was reported at any time point. Potential benefit of IAC injections in the hip joint has also been demonstrated [52].

ACR recommend intraarticular hyaluronic acid derivatives (IAHA) as an option for monoarticular large joint osteoarthritis in patients at risk for adverse effects of NSAIDs [10]. This option can be appealing for some older people. In osteoarthritis of the knee, a Cochrane review has reported that the efficacy of IAHA derivatives is comparable with NSAID [53]. These agents also have a longer lasting effect than IAC, peaking at 5-13 weeks. In practice, these agents may be effective in some patients but currently there is no means of identifying patients who will respond. Among older people, IAHA are options to try in patients with a single or a few large symptomatic joints and those who are too frail for surgery.

COMPLEMENTARY AGENTS

Glucosamine and chondroitin are available in many different formulations. As these preparations are unregulated, the actual content of glucosamine and chondroitin can vary from 0% to 115% of the labelled amount [54]. In a Cochrane systematic review of 15 RCTs, glucosamine sulphate was minimally effective for pain relief and no improvement in physical function or stiffness was found [55]. The efficacy of glucosamine and/or chondroitin is still controversial. In addition, these agents can be quite expensive but appear to be safe.

Fish oil use for osteoarthritis is gaining popularity despite the lack of evidence to support its efficacy, in contrast to rheumatoid arthritis. The components in fish oil, eicosapentaenoic acid and docosahexaenoic acid, have been found to reduce expression of degradative enzymes and inflammatory cytokines in in-vitro cartilage models of osteoarthritis [56, 57].

Many other nutritional and herbal supplements such as ginger extracts, methylsulfonylmethane and s-adenosylmethionine, have been reported anecdotally to decrease pain but all of these agents are unregulated [58, 59].

JOINT REPLACEMENT SURGERY

Many older patients who have severe symptomatic osteoarthritis may choose to undergo total hip arthroplasty (THA) or total knee arthroplasty (TKA) for long-term pain relief, functional and quality of life improvement. Several studies have shown beneficial outcomes after joint replacement surgery among older people [60, 61]. Patients who were at least 75 years old at the time of surgery improved their preoperative quality of life scores on the SF-36 to levels comparable to an age-matched nonsurgical group [60]. Another study demonstrates that elective THA and TKA in patients at least 80 years old had markedly improved postoperative knee and hip scores comparable to younger patients [61]. Therefore, age *per se* is not a barrier to hip and knee arthroplasty surgery in older people because postoperative outcomes mostly are correlated with preoperative comorbidities [62]. More importantly, preoperative planning ought to be an integral part of the assessment for THA and TKA surgery. The general goal is to identify and treat any conditions previously undiagnosed and to optimize known medical problems to reduce preoperative risk. Furthermore, there is a general trend that surgical approaches used in THA and TKA are less invasive in order to minimize soft tissue trauma, blood loss, and operative time.

Despite the best efforts in component design, patient selection, and preoperative and postoperative precautions in TKA and THA, complications still can occur. Intraoperative complications such as fat embolism, nerve injury (sciatic or common peroneal nerve) with resultant foot drop, vascular injury during THA and TKA are rare. Postoperative complications typically encountered after THA and TKA are venous thromboembolism, infections, dislocation, and periprosthetic fractures.

Venous thromboembolism, deep venous thrombosis (DVT) and pulmonary embolism (PE), are the most common complication after THA and TKA. Without effective postoperative prophylaxis, venous thromboembolism is reported to occur in more than 50% of patients who undergo THA or TKA [62]. It is approximately three times more likely in patients who have TKA compared with THA [63]. Older patients who are obese are particularly at risk for having adverse thromboembolic events after THA, with a mortality rate of 1.7% [64]. Similarly, the risk for fatal PE after TKA without thromboprophylaxis is 0.4% [65]. DVT alone causes significant morbidity in older patients as it leads to chronic venous insufficiency or post-thrombotic syndrome. There is a high incidence of post-thrombotic syndrome in patients after THA and TKA, approaching almost 100% at 10 years after the first DVT [66].

FUTURE RESEARCH

Two new pharmacological therapies are under investigation for osteoarthritis including blockade of interleukin-1 (IL1) and inhibition of nerve growth factor (NGF). The evaluation of intraarticular IL1 antagonist in osteoarthritis is still at its infancy [67]. Further evaluation of this agent is still required. Tanezumab, a humanized anti-NGF monoclonal antibody, has been evaluated in a randomized-controlled trial of 450 surgical candidates with knee osteoarthritis refractory to non-opiate analgesics [68]. This study demonstrated significant reduction in pain in tanezumab group compared to placebo. However this trial was discontinued because of an increase in the need for TKA in the tanezumab arm for reasons that are unclear.

Drugs targeting bone remodelling such as strontium ranelate, are also under investigation for use in osteoarthritis. RCTs have found strontium ranelate to reduce pain and radiological progression of osteoarthritis [69, 70]. However, long term studies are required to determine the safety of strontium ranelate in light of emerging data on cardiovascular risks [71].

New improvements to joint arthroplasty related to minimally invasive and computer-assisted navigation surgery techniques are promising [72, 73]. Outcomes of these newer techniques will need to be evaluated further in the older population.

CONCLUSION

The approach to management of osteoarthritis in older people needs to take into consideration the many factors that contribute to pain, functional decline and progression of disease. When treating pain related to osteoarthritis, non-pharmacological approaches including physical activity should always be incorporated into the management strategy that involves pharmacological agents. Use of topical and/or intraarticular agents should be included to minimize systemic adverse effects of oral analgesics. In older patients with severe osteoarthritis responding poorly to analgesics, total joint arthroplasty is the most effective intervention for those who are fit for surgery. There is a need for better therapeutic interventions for osteoarthritis. Further research is required to develop effective treatment for older patients with severe osteoarthritis who are not suitable candidates for surgical treatment.

CONFLICT OF INTEREST

The author confirms that author has no conflict of interest to declare for this publication.

ACKNOWLEDGEMENTS

Declared none.

KEY POINTS

- Osteoarthritis is a leading cause of pain and functional decline in older people.
- Nonpharmacological measures have an important role in the management of osteoarthritis-related pain and disability in the older population if medication adverse effects and polypharmacy are to be avoided.
- Pharmacological treatment gives mild-to-moderate pain relief in osteoarthritis but their long-term efficacy and safety in older people remain undetermined
- In older patients with severe osteoarthritis of the hips or knees responding poorly to analgesics, total joint arthroplasty is the most effective intervention for those who are fit for surgery.

REFERENCES

[1] Chodosh J, Morton SC, Mojica W, *et al.* Meta-analysis: chronic disease self-management programs for older adults. Ann Intern Med 2005; 143(6): 427-38. [http://dx.doi.org/10.7326/0003-4819-143-6-200509200-00007] [PMID: 16172441]

[2] Guccione AA, Felson DT, Anderson JJ, *et al.* The effects of specific medical conditions on the

functional limitations of elders in the Framingham Study. Am J Public Health 1994; 84(3): 351-8. [http://dx.doi.org/10.2105/AJPH.84.3.351] [PMID: 8129049]

[3] Bijlsma JW, Berenbaum F, Lafeber FP. Osteoarthritis: an update with relevance for clinical practice. Lancet 2011; 377(9783): 2115-26. [http://dx.doi.org/10.1016/S0140-6736(11)60243-2] [PMID: 21684382]

[4] Leveille SG, Fried L, Guralnik JM. Disabling symptoms: what do older women report? J Gen Intern Med 2002; 17(10): 766-73. [http://dx.doi.org/10.1046/j.1525-1497.2002.20229.x] [PMID: 12390552]

[5] Pharmacological management of persistent pain in older persons. J Am Geriatr Soc 2009; 57(8): 1331-46. [http://dx.doi.org/10.1111/j.1532-5415.2009.02376.x] [PMID: 19573219]

[6] Reid MC, Bennett DA, Chen WG, *et al.* Improving the pharmacologic management of pain in older adults: identifying the research gaps and methods to address them. Pain Med 2011; 12(9): 1336-57. [http://dx.doi.org/10.1111/j.1526-4637.2011.01211.x] [PMID: 21834914]

[7] Sharma L, Song J, Felson DT, Cahue S, Shamiyeh E, Dunlop DD. The role of knee alignment in disease progression and functional decline in knee osteoarthritis. JAMA 2001; 286(2): 188-95. [http://dx.doi.org/10.1001/jama.286.2.188] [PMID: 11448282]

[8] Altman R, Alarcón G, Appelrouth D, *et al.* The American College of Rheumatology criteria for the classification and reporting of osteoarthritis of the hip. Arthritis Rheum 1991; 34(5): 505-14. [http://dx.doi.org/10.1002/art.1780340502] [PMID: 2025304]

[9] Hannan MT, Felson DT, Pincus T. Analysis of the discordance between radiographic changes and knee pain in osteoarthritis of the knee. J Rheumatol 2000; 27(6): 1513-7. [PMID: 10852280]

[10] Recommendations for the medical management of osteoarthritis of the hip and knee: 2000 update. Arthritis Rheum 2000; 43(9): 1905-15. [http://dx.doi.org/10.1002/1529-0131(200009)43:9<1905::AID-ANR1>3.0.CO;2-P] [PMID: 11014340]

[11] Zhang W, Moskowitz RW, Nuki G, *et al.* OARSI recommendations for the management of hip and knee osteoarthritis, Part II: OARSI evidence-based, expert consensus guidelines. Osteoarthritis Cartilage 2008; 16(2): 137-62. [http://dx.doi.org/10.1016/j.joca.2007.12.013] [PMID: 18279766]

[12] Kerrigan DC, Lelas JL, Goggins J, Merriman GJ, Kaplan RJ, Felson DT. Effectiveness of a lateral-wedge insole on knee varus torque in patients with knee osteoarthritis. Arch Phys Med Rehabil 2002; 83(7): 889-93. [http://dx.doi.org/10.1053/apmr.2002.33225] [PMID: 12098144]

[13] Maillefert JF, Hudry C, Baron G, *et al.* Laterally elevated wedged insoles in the treatment of medial knee osteoarthritis: a prospective randomized controlled study. Osteoarthritis Cartilage 2001; 9(8): 738-45. [http://dx.doi.org/10.1053/joca.2001.0470] [PMID: 11795993]

[14] Pham T, Maillefert JF, Hudry C, *et al.* Laterally elevated wedged insoles in the treatment of medial

knee osteoarthritis. A two-year prospective randomized controlled study. Osteoarthritis Cartilage 2004; 12(1): 46-55.
[http://dx.doi.org/10.1016/j.joca.2003.08.011] [PMID: 14697682]

[15] Warden SJ, Hinman RS, Watson MA Jr, Avin KG, Bialocerkowski AE, Crossley KM. Patellar taping and bracing for the treatment of chronic knee pain: a systematic review and meta-analysis. Arthritis Rheum 2008; 59(1): 73-83.
[http://dx.doi.org/10.1002/art.23242] [PMID: 18163413]

[16] van Baar ME, Assendelft WJ, Dekker J, Oostendorp RA, Bijlsma JW. Effectiveness of exercise therapy in patients with osteoarthritis of the hip or knee: a systematic review of randomized clinical trials. Arthritis Rheum 1999; 42(7): 1361-9.
[http://dx.doi.org/10.1002/1529-0131(199907)42:7<1361::AID-ANR9>3.0.CO;2-9] [PMID: 10403263]

[17] Jansen MJ, Viechtbauer W, Lenssen AF, Hendriks EJ, de Bie RA. Strength training alone, exercise therapy alone, and exercise therapy with passive manual mobilisation each reduce pain and disability in people with knee osteoarthritis: a systematic review. J Physiother 2011; 57(1): 11-20.
[http://dx.doi.org/10.1016/S1836-9553(11)70002-9] [PMID: 21402325]

[18] Felson DT, Zhang Y. An update on the epidemiology of knee and hip osteoarthritis with a view to prevention. Arthritis Rheum 1998; 41(8): 1343-55.
[http://dx.doi.org/10.1002/1529-0131(199808)41:8<1343::AID-ART3>3.0.CO;2-9] [PMID: 9704632]

[19] Hunter DJ. Lower extremity osteoarthritis management needs a paradigm shift. Br J Sports Med 2011; 45(4): 283-8.
[http://dx.doi.org/10.1136/bjsm.2010.081117] [PMID: 21297174]

[20] Christensen R, Bartels EM, Astrup A, Bliddal H. Effect of weight reduction in obese patients diagnosed with knee osteoarthritis: a systematic review and meta-analysis. Ann Rheum Dis 2007; 66(4): 433-9.
[http://dx.doi.org/10.1136/ard.2006.065904] [PMID: 17204567]

[21] Miller SL, Wolfe RR. The danger of weight loss in the elderly. J Nutr Health Aging 2008; 12(7): 487-91.
[http://dx.doi.org/10.1007/BF02982710] [PMID: 18615231]

[22] Yu SP, Hunter DJ. Managing osteoarthritis. Aust Prescr 2015; 38(4): 115-9.
[PMID: 26648637]

[23] Bjordal JM, Klovning A, Ljunggren AE, Slørdal L. Short-term efficacy of pharmacotherapeutic interventions in osteoarthritic knee pain: A meta-analysis of randomised placebo-controlled trials. Eur J Pain 2007; 11(2): 125-38.
[http://dx.doi.org/10.1016/j.ejpain.2006.02.013] [PMID: 16682240]

[24] Geba GP, Weaver AL, Polis AB, Dixon ME, Schnitzer TJ. Efficacy of rofecoxib, celecoxib, and acetaminophen in osteoarthritis of the knee: a randomized trial. JAMA 2002; 287(1): 64-71.
[http://dx.doi.org/10.1001/jama.287.1.64] [PMID: 11754710]

[25] Spiegel BM, Farid M, Dulai GS, Gralnek IM, Kanwal F. Comparing rates of dyspepsia with Coxibs *vs* NSAID+PPI: a meta-analysis. Am J Med 2006; 119(5): 448.e27-36.
[http://dx.doi.org/10.1016/j.amjmed.2005.11.020] [PMID: 16651060]

[26] McGettigan P, Henry D. Cardiovascular risk and inhibition of cyclooxygenase: a systematic review of the observational studies of selective and nonselective inhibitors of cyclooxygenase 2. JAMA 2006; 296(13): 1633-44.
[http://dx.doi.org/10.1001/jama.296.13.jrv60011] [PMID: 16968831]

[27] Chou R, McDonagh MS, Nakamoto E, Griffin J. Analgesics for Osteoarthritis: An Update of the 2006 Comparative Effectiveness Review Rockville (MD). US: Agency for Healthcare Research and Quality 2011.AHRQ Comparative Effectiveness Reviews

[28] Luyten FP, Geusens P, Malaise M, *et al.* A prospective randomised multicentre study comparing continuous and intermittent treatment with celecoxib in patients with osteoarthritis of the knee or hip. Ann Rheum Dis 2007; 66(1): 99-106.
[http://dx.doi.org/10.1136/ard.2006.052308] [PMID: 16815864]

[29] McAlindon TE, Bannuru RR, Sullivan MC, *et al.* OARSI guidelines for the non-surgical management of knee osteoarthritis. Osteoarthritis Cartilage 2014; 22(3): 363-88.
[http://dx.doi.org/10.1016/j.joca.2014.01.003] [PMID: 24462672]

[30] Jevsevar DS, Brown GA, Jones DL, Matzkin EG, Manner PA, Mooar P, *et al.* The American Academy of Orthopaedic Surgeons evidence-based guideline on: treatment of osteoarthritis of the knee. J Bone Joint Surg 2013; 95(20): 1885-6.

[31] Machado GC, Maher CG, Ferreira PH, *et al.* Efficacy and safety of paracetamol for spinal pain and osteoarthritis: systematic review and meta-analysis of randomised placebo controlled trials. BMJ 2015; 350: h1225.
[http://dx.doi.org/10.1136/bmj.h1225] [PMID: 25828856]

[32] Miceli-Richard C, Le Bars M, Schmidely N, Dougados M. Paracetamol in osteoarthritis of the knee. Ann Rheum Dis 2004; 63(8): 923-30.
[http://dx.doi.org/10.1136/ard.2003.017236] [PMID: 15249319]

[33] Craig DG, Bates CM, Davidson JS, Martin KG, Hayes PC, Simpson KJ. Staggered overdose pattern and delay to hospital presentation are associated with adverse outcomes following paracetamol-induced hepatotoxicity. Br J Clin Pharmacol 2012; 73(2): 285-94.
[http://dx.doi.org/10.1111/j.1365-2125.2011.04067.x] [PMID: 22106945]

[34] Chan AT, Manson JE, Albert CM, *et al.* Nonsteroidal antiinflammatory drugs, acetaminophen, and the risk of cardiovascular events. Circulation 2006; 113(12): 1578-87.
[http://dx.doi.org/10.1161/CIRCULATIONAHA.105.595793] [PMID: 16534006]

[35] Rahme E, Barkun A, Nedjar H, Gaugris S, Watson D. Hospitalizations for upper and lower GI events associated with traditional NSAIDs and acetaminophen among the elderly in Quebec, Canada. Am J Gastroenterol 2008; 103(4): 872-82.
[http://dx.doi.org/10.1111/j.1572-0241.2008.01811.x] [PMID: 18371130]

[36] Cepeda MS, Camargo F, Zea C, Valencia L. Tramadol for osteoarthritis: a systematic review and metaanalysis. J Rheumatol 2007; 34(3): 543-55.
[PMID: 17343302]

[37] Vorsanger G, Xiang J, Jordan D, Farrell J. Post hoc analysis of a randomized, double-blind, placebo-controlled efficacy and tolerability study of tramadol extended release for the treatment of

osteoarthritis pain in geriatric patients. Clin Ther 2007; 29 (Suppl.): 2520-35. [http://dx.doi.org/10.1016/j.clinthera.2007.12.009] [PMID: 18164919]

[38] Chappell AS, Desaiah D, Liu-Seifert H, *et al.* A double-blind, randomized, placebo-controlled study of the efficacy and safety of duloxetine for the treatment of chronic pain due to osteoarthritis of the knee. Pain Pract 2011; 11(1): 33-41. [http://dx.doi.org/10.1111/j.1533-2500.2010.00401.x] [PMID: 20602715]

[39] Frakes EP, Risser RC, Ball TD, Hochberg MC, Wohlreich MM. Duloxetine added to oral nonsteroidal anti-inflammatory drugs for treatment of knee pain due to osteoarthritis: results of a randomized, double-blind, placebo-controlled trial. Curr Med Res Opin 2011; 27(12): 2361-72. [http://dx.doi.org/10.1185/03007995.2011.633502] [PMID: 22017192]

[40] da Costa BR, Nüesch E, Kasteler R, *et al.* Oral or transdermal opioids for osteoarthritis of the knee or hip. Cochrane Database Syst Rev 2014; 9: CD003115. [PMID: 25229835]

[41] Nüesch E, Rutjes AW, Husni E, Welch V, Jüni P. Oral or transdermal opioids for osteoarthritis of the knee or hip. Cochrane Database Syst Rev 2009; (4): CD003115. [PMID: 19821302]

[42] Solomon DH, Rassen JA, Glynn RJ, Lee J, Levin R, Schneeweiss S. The comparative safety of analgesics in older adults with arthritis. Arch Intern Med 2010; 170(22): 1968-76. [http://dx.doi.org/10.1001/archinternmed.2010.391] [PMID: 21149752]

[43] Mason L, Moore RA, Derry S, Edwards JE, McQuay HJ. Systematic review of topical capsaicin for the treatment of chronic pain. BMJ 2004; 328(7446): 991. [http://dx.doi.org/10.1136/bmj.38042.506748.EE] [PMID: 15033881]

[44] Lin J, Zhang W, Jones A, Doherty M. Efficacy of topical non-steroidal anti-inflammatory drugs in the treatment of osteoarthritis: meta-analysis of randomised controlled trials. BMJ 2004; 329(7461): 324. [http://dx.doi.org/10.1136/bmj.38159.639028.7C] [PMID: 15286056]

[45] Biswal S, Medhi B, Pandhi P. Longterm efficacy of topical nonsteroidal antiinflammatory drugs in knee osteoarthritis: metaanalysis of randomized placebo controlled clinical trials. J Rheumatol 2006; 33(9): 1841-4. [PMID: 16960944]

[46] Tugwell PS, Wells GA, Shainhouse JZ. Equivalence study of a topical diclofenac solution (pennsaid) compared with oral diclofenac in symptomatic treatment of osteoarthritis of the knee: a randomized controlled trial. J Rheumatol 2004; 31(10): 2002-12. [PMID: 15468367]

[47] Simon LS, Grierson LM, Naseer Z, Bookman AA, Zev Shainhouse J. Efficacy and safety of topical diclofenac containing dimethyl sulfoxide (DMSO) compared with those of topical placebo, DMSO vehicle and oral diclofenac for knee osteoarthritis. Pain 2009; 143(3): 238-45. [http://dx.doi.org/10.1016/j.pain.2009.03.008] [PMID: 19380203]

[48] Peniston JH, Gold MS, Wieman MS, Alwine LK. Long-term tolerability of topical diclofenac sodium 1% gel for osteoarthritis in seniors and patients with comorbidities. Clin Interv Aging 2012; 7: 517-23. [http://dx.doi.org/10.2147/CIA.S35416] [PMID: 23204844]

[49] Gammaitoni AR, Galer BS, Onawola R, Jensen MP, Argoff CE. Lidocaine patch 5% and its positive impact on pain qualities in osteoarthritis: results of a pilot 2-week, open-label study using the Neuropathic Pain Scale. Curr Med Res Opin 2004; 20 (Suppl. 2): S13-9. [http://dx.doi.org/10.1185/030079904X12951] [PMID: 15563742]

[50] Burch F, Codding C, Patel N, Sheldon E. Lidocaine patch 5% improves pain, stiffness, and physical function in osteoarthritis pain patients. A prospective, multicenter, open-label effectiveness trial. Osteoarthritis Cartilage 2004; 12(3): 253-5. [http://dx.doi.org/10.1016/j.joca.2003.10.007] [PMID: 14972343]

[51] Bellamy N, Campbell J, Robinson V, Gee T, Bourne R, Wells G. Intraarticular corticosteroid for treatment of osteoarthritis of the knee. Cochrane Database Syst Rev 2006; (2): CD005328. [PMID: 16625636]

[52] Micu MC, Bogdan GD, Fodor D. Steroid injection for hip osteoarthritis: efficacy under ultrasound guidance. Rheumatology (Oxford) 2010; 49(8): 1490-4. [http://dx.doi.org/10.1093/rheumatology/keq030] [PMID: 20338889]

[53] Bellamy N, Campbell J, Robinson V, Gee T, Bourne R, Wells G. Viscosupplementation for the treatment of osteoarthritis of the knee. Cochrane Database Syst Rev 2006; (2): CD005321. [PMID: 16625635]

[54] Biggee BA, Blinn CM, McAlindon TE, Nuite M, Silbert JE. Low levels of human serum glucosamine after ingestion of glucosamine sulphate relative to capability for peripheral effectiveness. Ann Rheum Dis 2006; 65(2): 222-6. [http://dx.doi.org/10.1136/ard.2005.036368] [PMID: 16079170]

[55] Towheed TE, Maxwell L, Anastassiades TP, *et al.* Glucosamine therapy for treating osteoarthritis. Cochrane Database Syst Rev 2005; (2): CD002946. [PMID: 15846645]

[56] Cleland LG, James MJ. Osteoarthritis. Omega-3 fatty acids and synovitis in osteoarthritic knees. Nat Rev Rheumatol 2012; 8(6): 314-5. [http://dx.doi.org/10.1038/nrrheum.2012.60] [PMID: 22508432]

[57] Lopez HL. Nutritional interventions to prevent and treat osteoarthritis. Part I: focus on fatty acids and macronutrients. PM R 2012; 4(5) (Suppl.): S145-54. [http://dx.doi.org/10.1016/j.pmrj.2012.02.022] [PMID: 22632694]

[58] Ernst E. Complementary or alternative therapies for osteoarthritis. Nat Clin Pract Rheumatol 2006; 2(2): 74-80. [http://dx.doi.org/10.1038/ncprheum0093] [PMID: 16932660]

[59] Lopez HL. Nutritional interventions to prevent and treat osteoarthritis. Part II: focus on micronutrients and supportive nutraceuticals. PM R 2012; 4(5) (Suppl.): S155-68. [http://dx.doi.org/10.1016/j.pmrj.2012.02.023] [PMID: 22632695]

[60] March LM, Cross MJ, Lapsley H, *et al.* Outcomes after hip or knee replacement surgery for osteoarthritis. A prospective cohort study comparing patients' quality of life before and after surgery with age-related population norms. Med J Aust 1999; 171(5): 235-8. [PMID: 10495753]

[61] Brander VA, Malhotra S, Jet J, Heinemann AW, Stulberg SD. Outcome of hip and knee arthroplasty in persons aged 80 years and older. Clin Orthop Res 1997; pp. 67-78.

[62] St Clair SF, Higuera C, Krebs V, Tadross NA, Dumpe J, Barsoum WK. Hip and knee arthroplasty in the geriatric population. Clin Geriatr Med 2006; 22(3): 515-33. [http://dx.doi.org/10.1016/j.cger.2006.04.004] [PMID: 16860243]

[63] Fujita S, Hirota S, Oda T, Kato Y, Tsukamoto Y, Fuji T. Deep venous thrombosis after total hip or total knee arthroplasty in patients in Japan. Clin Orthop Res 2000; pp. 168-74.

[64] White RH, Gettner S, Newman JM, Trauner KB, Romano PS. Predictors of rehospitalization for symptomatic venous thromboembolism after total hip arthroplasty. N Engl J Med 2000; 343(24): 1758-64. [http://dx.doi.org/10.1056/NEJM200012143432403] [PMID: 11114314]

[65] Ansari S, Warwick D, Ackroyd CE, Newman JH. Incidence of fatal pulmonary embolism after 1,390 knee arthroplasties without routine prophylactic anticoagulation, except in high-risk cases. J Arthroplasty 1997; 12(6): 599-602. [http://dx.doi.org/10.1016/S0883-5403(97)90131-5] [PMID: 9306209]

[66] Edelsberg J, Ollendorf D, Oster G. Venous thromboembolism following major orthopedic surgery: review of epidemiology and economics. Am J Health Syst Pharm 2001; 58 (Suppl. 2): S4-S13. [PMID: 11715837]

[67] Chevalier X, Goupille P, Beaulieu AD, *et al.* Intraarticular injection of anakinra in osteoarthritis of the knee: a multicenter, randomized, double-blind, placebo-controlled study. Arthritis Rheum 2009; 61(3): 344-52. [http://dx.doi.org/10.1002/art.24096] [PMID: 19248129]

[68] Lane NE, Schnitzer TJ, Birbara CA, *et al.* Tanezumab for the treatment of pain from osteoarthritis of the knee. N Engl J Med 2010; 363(16): 1521-31. [http://dx.doi.org/10.1056/NEJMoa0901510] [PMID: 20942668]

[69] Reginster JY, Badurski J, Bellamy N, *et al.* Efficacy and safety of strontium ranelate in the treatment of knee osteoarthritis: results of a double-blind, randomised placebo-controlled trial. Ann Rheum Dis 2013; 72(2): 179-86. [http://dx.doi.org/10.1136/annrheumdis-2012-202231] [PMID: 23117245]

[70] Bruyère O, Reginster JY, Bellamy N, Chapurlat R, Richette P, Cooper C. Clinically meaningful effect of strontium ranelate on symptoms in knee osteoarthritis: a responder analysis. Rheumatology (Oxford) 2014; 53(8): 1457-64. [http://dx.doi.org/10.1093/rheumatology/keu018] [PMID: 24667161]

[71] Abrahamsen B, Grove EL, Vestergaard P. Nationwide registry-based analysis of cardiovascular risk factors and adverse outcomes in patients treated with strontium ranelate. Osteoporos Int 2014; 25(2): 757-62. [http://dx.doi.org/10.1007/s00198-013-2469-4] [PMID: 24322475]

[72] Bonutti PM, Seyler TM, Kester M, McMahon M, Mont MA. Minimally invasive revision total knee arthroplasty. Clin Orthop Relat Res 2006; 446: 69-75. [http://dx.doi.org/10.1097/01.blo.0000218728.52214.ac] [PMID: 16672874]

[73] Chauhan SK, Scott RG, Breidahl W, Beaver RJ. Computer-assisted knee arthroplasty *versus* a conventional jig-based technique. A randomised, prospective trial. J Bone Joint Surg Br 2004; 86(3): 372-7.
[http://dx.doi.org/10.1302/0301-620X.86B3.14643] [PMID: 15125124]

CHAPTER 10

Towards Unbreakable Old Bones: Osteoporosis in Older Adults

Kareeann Sok Fun Khow[1,*], Tuck Yean Yong[2]

[1] *Aged and Extended Care Services, The Queen Elizabeth Hospital and Department of Medicine, University of Adelaide, Adelaide, South Australia, Australia*

[2] *Internal Medicine, Flinders Private Hospital, Flinders Drive, Bedford Park, South Australia 5042, Australia*

Abstract: Osteoporosis is characterised by bone demineralisation, reduction in bone mass and changes in bone micro-architecture or the presence of a fragility fracture. Osteoporosis is still frequently underdiagnosed and undertreated. Advancing age is a risk factor for underdiagnosis and undertreatment of osteoporosis. The goal of treatment is to reduce morbidity and mortality associated with the first fracture and prevent subsequent fractures. Osteoporosis management in older adults (≥65 years of age) must involve both non-pharmacological and pharmacological interventions. Beneficial non-pharmacological interventions include falls risk assessment and management, participation in exercise programs and the use of hip protectors. Pharmacological treatments including calcium, vitamin D, bisphosphonates, denosumab, strontium and teriparatide are generally safe for use in older people and significantly reduce fracture risk especially vertebral fractures. However the evidence is not as strong for reducing the risk in non-vertebral and hip fractures.

Keywords: Bisphosphonate, Bone loss, Calcium, Denosumab, Falls prevention, Fractures, Older people, Osteoclast, Osteoporosis, Parathyroid hormone, Strontium, Vitamin D.

* **Correspondence author Kareeann Sok Fun Khow:** Aged and Extended Care Service, The Queen Elizabeth Hospital, Woodville Road, Woodville, South Australia 5011, Australia; Tel: +61 8 8222 6000; Fax: +61 8 8222 8593; E-mail: kareeann.khow@adelaide.edu.au .

INTRODUCTION

Osteoporosis is characterised by the loss of bone mass and micro-architectural deterioration of bone resulting in enhanced bone fragility and increase in risk of fracture. Osteoporosis is closely linked with aging because as people age, bone resorption by osteoclasts is not fully restored with bone deposition by osteoblasts leading to bone loss. The prevalence of osteoporosis is increasing because of extended life expectancy and an ageing population.

Worldwide, epidemiological data have shown that the annual incidence of fragility fractures increases with age [1]. In Australia, approximately 75,000 fragility fractures occur annually which includes about 21,000 hip fractures [2]. Fragility fractures are associated with significant disability, mortality and costs [3]. The burden of fragility fractures is expected to rise with an ageing population [2, 4]. Worldwide, 85% of residents in aged care facilities (RACFs) are reported to have osteoporosis [5] and approximately 40% of all hip fractures occur in this population [6].

This chapter will review changes in the bone with increasing age, diagnosis of osteoporosis, prevention of fragility fractures in older people and advances in osteoporosis treatment.

CHANGES IN BONE AND GAIT STABILITY WITH AGING

The decline in cancellous bone mass in humans begins in the third decade while loss of cortical bone starts after 50 years of age [7]. In women, bone loss occurs at a faster rate after menopause because of skeletal involution associated with estrogen deficiency. The important pathogenetic mechanism in age-related bone loss appears to be impaired bone formation attributed to decline in osteoblast numbers. This deterioration is thought to be due to a decline in the number of mesenchymal stem cells, defective proliferation or differentiation of progenitor cells, or diversion of these progenitor cells toward the adipocyte lineage, and also to increased apoptosis [8].

Age-related bone loss is largely a result of senescence mechanisms that affect bone cell number and function. These mechanisms can relate to intrinsic senescence processes, alterations in endogenous anabolic factors and changes in local support [9, 10]. Intrinsic senescence mechanisms include telomere shortening, accumulation of oxidative stress, impairment in DNA repair and altered epigenetic processes that regulate gene expression [8]. Extrinsic mechanisms of bone senescence include deficiency in sex-hormone, decreased physical activity, nutritional deficiency and alcohol consumption or smoking [11]. Local disruptions include among others, altered signalling pathways and cell-cell communication as well as signal dysregulation in osteogenic niches [12].

Both trabecular and cortical bone are affected by these age-related changes. Based on its pathophysiology and affected regions, osteoporosis has been classified into two types: postmenopausal osteoporosis and senile osteoporosis.

DIAGNOSIS

Apart from fragility fracture being a characteristic feature of osteoporosis, diagnosis is dependent on bone mineral density (BMD) measurement with a dual-energy X-ray absorptiometry (DXA). For women, the World Health Organization (WHO) and International Osteoporosis Foundation (IOF) have identified four diagnostic groups for DXA which is used to guide treatment (Table **1**) [13].

Table 1. World Health Organisation and International Osteoporosis Foundation dual-energy X-ray absorptiometry assessment diagnostic categories.

Category	T-Score of Hip Bone Mineral Density
Normal	≥-1.0
Osteopenia (low bone mass)	<-1.0 and >-2.5
Osteoporosis	≤-2.5
Severe osteoporosis (established osteoporosis)	≤-2.5 and presence of at least one fragility fracture

T-score is the number of standard deviations below the mean value of the young healthy population.

Two risk assessment tools are available to facilitate the assessment of fracture risk in the community-dwelling population. The FRAX [14] and the Garvan [15] fracture risk assessment tools have been useful in identifying people at risk of osteoporosis and determining the threshold for treatment. However the applicability of these tools among residents of RACFs remains unknown.

STRATEGIES TO PREVENT FRAGILITY FRACTURES

In general, the aims of osteoporosis treatment are to reduce morbidity and mortality associated with the first fracture and to prevent further fractures. Osteoporosis management and fracture prevention in older people must focus on both non-pharmacological and pharmacological interventions.

Non-Pharmacological

Falls Prevention

Each year, falls occur in about 30% of people aged 50 years and above who live in the community and over 50% of those who live in RACFs [16]. Falls can result in any type of fracture in about 5% and hip fracture in 1-2% of events [17]. Therefore reducing falls is a high health care priority in an ageing population with high prevalence of osteoporosis. Falls are associated with identifiable risk factors such as unsteady gait, visual impairment, cognitive impairment and polypharmacy. Addressing these factors can significantly reduce falls. Furthermore, there is a growing body of evidence that supports falls prevention programs involving regular medication reviews, multidisciplinary interventions, environment modifications [18].

Exercise Programs

Muscle weakness and impaired balance are risk factors for falls. These factors are potentially preventable or modifiable with exercise. Exercise programs for older people living the community have been reported to reduce falls risk by 15-50% [19]. Balance exercise three times a week is one option which has been found to be effective in a meta-analysis of four falls prevention studies [20].

Hip Protectors

Hip protector is a method of redirecting the force and energy of a fall away from the hip and reduce the risk of hip fractures sustained as a consequence of a fall. Although studies have found variable outcomes with hip protectors, evidence supports their use when adherence to wearing them is adequate [21, 22].

Pharmacological

Pharmacological treatment of osteoporosis based on BMD assessment has been found to be cost-effective in older community populations [23, 24]. Current osteoporosis treatment can be categorised into three groups: antiresorptives, anabolics and dual action. Antiresorptives are agents that inhibit bone resorption, such as bisphosphonates, denosumab and cathepsin K inhibitors. Anabolic agents are those that induce bone formation such as analogue of parathyroid hormone and anti-sclerostin antibody [25]. Drugs with dual effects have the ability to reduce bone resorption and increase or maintain bone formation. An example of a treatment with dual effect is strontium ranelate. In general, selection of the most appropriate osteoporosis treatment should consider their likely potential benefit; optimal dose frequency and route of administration; potential adverse effects and patient tolerance; issues with adherence; cost effectiveness; and ability to prevent fractures. A systematic review of economic analyses for osteoporosis treatment have shown that despite methodological differences, models consistently show improved cost-effectiveness with advancing age, with treatment between the ages of 80 and 90 years emerging as cost-saving in nearly all models [26].

Calcium and Vitamin D Supplementation

Calcium and vitamin D supplementation are not a direct treatment but important co-adjuvants of any osteoporosis treatment. Dose of vitamin D should be aimed at maintaining serum levels >75 nmol/L, which is usually obtained with a regular dose of 1,000 IU/day [27]. The recommended dose of calcium supplementation is 1.2 g/day [28]. However, recent concerns about potential cardiovascular risks associated with calcium supplementation have changed the practice into highlighting the importance of dietary calcium and of reducing the recommended calcium dose by 50% [29]. Nevertheless, the majority of the major clinical trials testing osteoporosis treatments have included calcium and vitamin D as co-adjuvants and, therefore, adding them into any fracture prevention plan is usually standard [30]. Furthermore, vitamin D should be greater than 50 nmol/L before administration of bisphosphonates or denosumab to lower the risk of hypocalcaemia [31].

Oestrogen

Oestrogen initiated within 10 years of menopause prevents bone loss at the spine and hip [32]. Nonetheless, there are few prospective studies evaluating oestrogen replacement and fracture prevention in women 70 years and older [33]. The risks of long-term therapy with estrogens (*i.e.*, breast carcinoma, thromboembolism, cardiovascular events *etc.*) outweighs their benefits on fracture reduction [34]. Therefore and considering the safer alternatives available for the treatment of osteoporosis in elderly patients (particularly those at least 5-10 years post-menopausal), oestrogen therapy for osteoporosis is not recommended [35].

Bisphosphonate

Bisphosphonates have well-established anti-fracture efficacy in both old and peri-menopausal populations with osteoporosis [31]. Three oral bisphosphonate agents (alendronate, risedronate and ibandronate) and one intravenous (zoledronic acid) are commonly used. The effectiveness of these treatments in older women is summarized in (Table **2**). Alendronate has vertebral fracture reduction efficacy in postmenopausal women, in men, in glucocorticoid-induced osteoporosis and non-vertebral fracture reduction including hip fractures [36]. Similarly, risedronate reduce vertebral fractures, non-vertebral fractures, hip fractures in osteoporotic older women and glucocorticoid induced osteoporosis [37 - 39]. Both alendronate (70 mg) and risedronate (35 mg) are given weekly, whereas risedronate and ibandronate could also be administered monthly (150 mg).

Table 2. Summary of data on the efficacy of osteoporosis treatment in women aged 65 years and over.

Drug	**Primary Efficacy Analysis**			**Older Subgroup Analysis**			**Studies with a Significant Number of Older Subjects**
	VF	NVF	HF	VF	NVF	HF	
Alendronate	+	+*	+	+	NA	NA	Jamal S, *et al.* [36] Age ≥75 years VF risk = 0.62 (95% CI: 0.41-0.94)

(Table 2) contd.....

Drug	Primary Efficacy Analysis			Older Subgroup Analysis			Studies with a Significant Number of Older Subjects
	VF	NVF	HF	VF	NVF	HF	
Risedronate	+	+	+	+	-	+	Boonen S, *et al.* [38] Age ≥80 years VF risk = 0.56 (95% CI: 0.39-0.81) NVF risk = non-significant McClung M, *et al.* [37] Age 70-79 years HF risk = 0.6 (95% CI: 0.4-0.9) Age ≥80 years† HF risk = non-significant Masud T, *et al.* [39] Age 70-100 years‡ HF = 0.54 (95% CI: 0.32-0.91)
Zolendronate	+	+	+	+	+	-	Boonen S, *et al.* [55] Age ≥75 years Clinical VF risk = 0.34 (95% CI: 0.21-0.55) NVF risk = 0.73 (95% CI: 0.6-0.9) HF risk = 0.82 (95% CI: 0.56-1.2, p = 0.66)
Strontium ranelate	+	+	-	+	+	+§	Reginster J, *et al.* [47] Age ≥74 years; FN BMD ≤-2.5 §HF risk =0.64 (95% CI: 0.412-0.997) Seeman E, *et al.* [56] Age ≥80 years VF risk =0.68 (95% CI: 0.50-0.92) NVF risk =0.69 (95% CI: 0.52-0.92) HF risk =0.68 (95% CI: 0.42-1.10, p =NS)
Denosumab	+	+	+	+	NA	+	Boonen S, *et al.* [57] Age ≥75 years VF risk =0.68 (95% CI: 0.46-0.94) HF risk =0.38 (95% CI: 0.18-0.78)

*Not significant in FIT-1 and FIT-2 but significant in FOSIT (at 1 year).

†Subgroup of patients with one or more clinical risk factors for hip fracture or FN BMD ≤-4 or ≤-3 with hip axis length ≥11.1 cm.

‡Patients with established osteoporosis (FN BMD ≤-2.5 and one or more prevalent vertebral fractures

§Subgroup of patients with additional risk factor for fracture (FN BMD ≤-2.5).

+: Significant fracture risk reduction observed; -: Significant fracture risk reduction not observed; CI: confidence interval; FN BMD: Femoral neck bone mineral density T-score; HF: Hip fracture; NA: data unavailable; NVF: Nonvertebral fracture; VF: Vertebral fracture

Despite their effectiveness, these two medications have major limitations in terms of adherence due to their way of administration, which involves having an empty stomach, drinking a lot of water and standing upright for a specific period of time. Following these instructions is challenging particularly in older persons [40].

Zoledronic acid, an intravenous bisphosphonate, is also efficacious for reduction of vertebral, hip and non-vertebral fractures in both men and women and glucocorticoid-induced osteoporosis [41, 42]. An additional effect of zoledronic acid is a significant reduction in mortality (28%) within one year after hip fracture [43]. The mechanisms of this beneficial effect remain unclear. Zoledronate is administered yearly (5 mg), which assures 100% compliance with anti-fracture efficacy that could remain up to 3 years after the first dose [44].

An important limitation to the use of both oral and intravenous bisphosphonates in older people is that these drugs are contraindicated in patients with low glomerular filtration rate (GFR) (<35 mL/min), which narrows the spectrum of patients who can benefit from these treatments [3].

Although the effectiveness of bisphosphonates on fracture prevention is clearly demonstrated, there are recent reports of higher incidence of atypical fractures in patients taking bisphosphonates [45]. These atypical fractures, which have been associated with the strong inhibitory effect of bisphosphonates on bone turnover [46], are usually subtrochanteric and are associated with cortical thickening and periosteal tearing in patients on anti-resorptives for long periods of time. A recent panel of experts recognized that, although rare, atypical fractures are a side effect of these compounds and recommended a set of measures to identify patients at risk and to initiate appropriate and prompt preventive interventions [46].

Strontium Ranelate

Strontium ranelate reduces vertebral and non-vertebral fractures including hip in post-menopausal osteoporosis. Evidence from clinical trials suggests that it is effective in a wide range of patient profiles including for older women over the age of 80 years [3]. The antifracture efficacy of strontium ranelate has been shown to be independent of baseline severity of osteoporosis, bone turnover level or the presence of clinical risk factors [3]. Furthermore, the antifracture efficacy of strontium ranelate is sustained over 10 years [47]. Strontium is administered orally at a dose of 2 g/day dissolved in water. Due to its method and frequency of administration, adherence can be an issue in older people. Adverse effects of strontium include gastrointestinal symptoms such as nausea or diarrhoea and increased risk of venous thromboembolism and cardiovascular events, which are more prevalent in older persons [48].

Selective Oestrogen Receptor Modulator

Selective oestrogen receptor modulator (SERM) such as raloxifene has beneficial oestrogen-like effects on bone. A randomised controlled trial has shown that raloxifene reduces vertebral fractures and increases BMD in the spine and femoral neck [49]. However there is little evidence to suggest that raloxifene may prevent nonvertebral fractures. No study has evaluated the use of SERM in preventing osteoporosis-related fractures in older people.

Denosumab

Denosumab is a human monoclonal antibody to receptor activator of nuclear factor kappa-β ligand (RANKL). Denosumab blocks RANKL binding to RANK thus inhibiting the development and activity of osteoclasts [50]. Six monthly subcutaneous injections of denosumab for 36 months was shown to reduce the risk of new radiographic vertebral fractures by 68%, hip fractures by 40% and non-vertebral fractures by 20% in a mixed age cohort [51].

There was no increase in the risk of cancer and infection compared to placebo, however, the major concern about the long-term use of denosumab relates to its possible effects on the immune system, since RANKL is expressed not just on bone cells but also on immune cells, which could explain a significant increase in the occurrence of eczema and serious infections in the denosumab group compared with placebo [52].

The advantages of using denosumab in older persons include (a) improvement in adherence due to convenient biannual subcutaneous administration; (b) reversibility, because it targets RANKL and is not incorporated into the bone mineral; (c) lack of gastrointestinal side effects and (d) useful in patients with impaired kidney function, which is highly prevalent in older persons.

This last advantage is more evident in older persons in whom low glomerular filtration rate (GFR) is a common finding. In terms of adverse effects, there are recent reports of atypical fractures in patients treated with denosumab [53, 54] which will require ongoing vigilance by clinicians.

Human Recombinant Parathyroid Hormone

Two anabolic agents have been approved for the treatment of osteoporosis, teriparatide, a 1-34 amino acid fragment of human recombinant PTH [PTH (1-34)], and in Europe the full length PTH (1-84) molecule [25]. Teriparatide stimulates bone turnover. Teriparatide has been shown to reduce vertebral and non-vertebral fracture in post-menopausal women with osteoporosis [58, 59]. Compared to alendronate, teriparatide produced earlier and greater gains in BMD at the lumbar spine and total hip [25]. In addition, this drug was more effective in preventing new vertebral fractures [25]. Teriparatide is administered subcutaneously at a dose of 20 μg/day. Since it requires certain level of training, older persons could find this treatment as challenging. However, support services and education programs have facilitated patients' learning and have also increased compliance [60].

Other New Agents

There are two new classes of treatment for osteoporosis under clinical trial: Cathepsin K inhibitors such as odanacatib and anti-sclerostin antibody. Cathepsin K inhibitors target the resorption process and may not interfere with osteoclast stimulation of bone formation [61]. Phase I and II studies with odanacatib have shown that at 36 months, the drug achieves increases in BMD similar to zoledronate and denosumab [62 - 64]. However, compared to zolendronate and denosumab, the reduction in resorption markers is less with odanacatib but there is also smaller reduction in bone formation markers [61]. The anti-fracture effect of odanacatib is being tested in an ongoing randomized double-blind placebo-controlled clinical trial of 16,000 treatment naive post-menopausal women age 65 and above.

By inhibiting sclerostin, anti-sclerostin antibody should enhance osteoblastic function [65]. In a Phase II study of postmenopausal women with low bone mass, romosozumab, an anti-sclerostin antibody, was associated with increased bone mineral density and bone formation and with decreased bone resorption [66]. The role of these new agents in the treatment of osteoporosis in older people have not been explored.

MANAGING OSTEOPOROSIS IN RESIDENTS OF AGED CARE FACILITIES

Older people living in RACFs are at significantly higher risk of fragility fractures than those living in the community [6, 67]. For primary prevention of fractures among older people in RACFs, calcium and vitamin D should be prescribed, and multifactorial falls prevention implemented. On admission to RACFs, new residents should be screened for falls risk but there is as yet an assessment tool that is developed specifically for this population. Risk assessment should be repeated every 6 months or in the event of a fall. For secondary prevention, in addition to calcium, vitamin D and multifactorial falls prevention strategies, people living in RACFs should be treated with oral or intravenous bisphosphonates provided there is no contraindications [22].

Strontium ranelate is the only agent that has demonstrated a reduction in nonvertebral and hip fracture in high risk older female population but no study has assessed its effect in a RACF population [3, 47]. Teriparatide is not recommended for use as a first-line treatment and should only be reserved for specific indications such as contraindications or lack of response to other treatment modalities.

OSTEOPOROSIS AND MULTIPLE COMORBIDITIES

Kidney impairment is common among older people and this comorbidity is an important consideration in selecting the appropriate therapy for osteoporosis. Calcium concentration should be monitored in patients with kidney impairment who receive calcium supplement. Bisphosphonates are excreted mainly unchanged through the kidneys and should not be used in patients with GFR of <35 mL/min [3]. Strontium ranelate and teriparatide are also not recommended in people with GFR <30 mL/min [3].

Systemic corticosteroid therapy is one of the most common secondary causes of osteoporosis and its use is relatively common among older people for various clinical indications. Up to 30-50% of people treated with long-term corticosteroid treatment may sustain a fragility fracture and this risk rises to as high as 75% during the first three months [68]. Therefore bone health should be a priority in older people who are treated with long-term systemic corticosteroid therapy.

GAPS IN CURRENT EVIDENCE AND FUTURE RESEARCH

There is still a limited evidence for management of osteoporosis in older men with most published studies focusing on women only. In addition, evidence indicates that fracture prevention and osteoporosis treatment in older people at high fracture risk is less commonly practised than expected [69, 70]. Being a "silent" condition, patients will not consult their medical practitioner about their osteoporosis risk and clinicians rarely assess patients about the presence of risk factors for osteoporosis. There is opportunity for the care gap to be closed by raising awareness of this disease, implementing fracture liaison services and equipping clinicians with the necessary tools to prevent fractures in older people.

The current therapeutic choices for osteoporosis are limited to antiresorptives and anabolic agents. Most of these agents have either reached a therapeutic plateau in terms of their fracture prevention effect or have shown unexpected side effects that could limit their long-term use. Therefore new therapeutic targets are being explored and their potential benefits in older people with osteoporosis will need to be investigated.

CONCLUSION

As the population ages, osteoporosis and associated fragility fractures will continue to be an important public health issue. Identifying older people at risk of osteoporosis and falls is a crucial step to prevent fragility fractures. Nonpharmacological and pharmacological interventions have complementary roles in the management of osteoporosis. Evidence supports the use of bisphosphonates, strontium renolate or denosumab in older people as a safe approach to reduce the risk of fractures.

CONFLICT OF INTEREST

The author confirms that author has no conflict of interest to declare for this publication.

ACKNOWLEDGEMENTS

Declared none.

KEY POINTS

- Osteoporosis and fragility fractures are highly prevalent in older people, aged ≥65 years.
- Osteoporosis is underdiagnosed and undertreated in older people.
- Osteoporosis management and prevention of fragility fractures in older people must involve both non-pharmacological and pharmacological approaches.
- Falls risk assessment and prevention, and exercise programs are beneficial non-pharmacological approaches.
- Therapies such as calcium, vitamin D, bisphosphonates, strontium and denosumab are safe in older people and reduce fractures, especially vertebral fractures.

REFERENCES

[1] Felsenberg D, Silman AJ, Lunt M, *et al.* Incidence of vertebral fracture in Europe: results from the European Prospective Osteoporosis Study (EPOS). J Bone Miner Res 2002; 17(4): 716-24. [http://dx.doi.org/10.1359/jbmr.2002.17.4.716] [PMID: 11918229]

[2] Sanders KM, Seeman E, Ugoni AM, *et al.* Age- and gender-specific rate of fractures in Australia: a population-based study. Osteoporos Int 1999; 10(3): 240-7. [http://dx.doi.org/10.1007/s001980050222] [PMID: 10525717]

[3] Inderjeeth CA, Foo AC, Lai MM, Glendenning P. Efficacy and safety of pharmacological agents in managing osteoporosis in the old old: review of the evidence. Bone 2009; 44(5): 744-51. [http://dx.doi.org/10.1016/j.bone.2008.12.003] [PMID: 19130909]

[4] Jones G, Nguyen T, Sambrook PN, Kelly PJ, Gilbert C, Eisman JA. Symptomatic fracture incidence in elderly men and women: the Dubbo Osteoporosis Epidemiology Study (DOES). Osteoporos Int 1994; 4(5): 277-82. [http://dx.doi.org/10.1007/BF01623352] [PMID: 7812076]

[5] Parikh S, Avorn J, Solomon DH. Pharmacological management of osteoporosis in nursing home populations: a systematic review. J Am Geriatr Soc 2009; 57(2): 327-34. [http://dx.doi.org/10.1111/j.1532-5415.2008.02119.x] [PMID: 19207148]

[6] Norton R, Campbell AJ, Reid IR, *et al.* Residential status and risk of hip fracture. Age Ageing 1999; 28(2): 135-9.
[http://dx.doi.org/10.1093/ageing/28.2.135] [PMID: 10350409]

[7] Riggs BL, Melton LJ, Robb RA, *et al.* A population-based assessment of rates of bone loss at multiple skeletal sites: evidence for substantial trabecular bone loss in young adult women and men. J Bone Miner Res 2008; 23(2): 205-14.
[http://dx.doi.org/10.1359/jbmr.071020] [PMID: 17937534]

[8] Kassem M, Marie PJ. Senescence-associated intrinsic mechanisms of osteoblast dysfunctions. Aging Cell 2011; 10(2): 191-7.
[http://dx.doi.org/10.1111/j.1474-9726.2011.00669.x] [PMID: 21210937]

[9] Marie PJ. Bone cell senescence: mechanisms and perspectives. J Bone Miner Res 2014; 29(6): 1311-21.
[http://dx.doi.org/10.1002/jbmr.2190] [PMID: 24496911]

[10] Demontiero O, Vidal C, Duque G. Aging and bone loss: new insights for the clinician. Ther Adv Musculoskelet Dis 2012; 4(2): 61-76.
[http://dx.doi.org/10.1177/1759720X11430858] [PMID: 22870496]

[11] Marie PJ, Kassem M. Extrinsic mechanisms involved in age-related defective bone formation. J Clin Endocrinol Metab 2011; 96(3): 600-9.
[http://dx.doi.org/10.1210/jc.2010-2113] [PMID: 21209032]

[12] Genetos DC, Zhou Z, Li Z, Donahue HJ. Age-related changes in gap junctional intercellular communication in osteoblastic cells. J Orthop Res 2012; 30(12): 1979-84.
[http://dx.doi.org/10.1002/jor.22172] [PMID: 22696456]

[13] Kanis JA, Glüer CC. An update on the diagnosis and assessment of osteoporosis with densitometry. Committee of Scientific Advisors, International Osteoporosis Foundation. Osteoporos Int 2000; 11(3): 192-202.
[http://dx.doi.org/10.1007/s001980050281] [PMID: 10824234]

[14] Kanis JA, Oden A, Johansson H, Borgström F, Ström O, McCloskey E. FRAX and its applications to clinical practice. Bone 2009; 44(5): 734-43.
[http://dx.doi.org/10.1016/j.bone.2009.01.373] [PMID: 19195497]

[15] Nguyen ND, Frost SA, Center JR, Eisman JA, Nguyen TV. Development of prognostic nomograms for individualizing 5-year and 10-year fracture risks. Osteoporos Int 2008; 19(10): 1431-44.
[http://dx.doi.org/10.1007/s00198-008-0588-0] [PMID: 18324342]

[16] Kannus P, Sievänen H, Palvanen M, Järvinen T, Parkkari J. Prevention of falls and consequent injuries in elderly people. Lancet 2005; 366(9500): 1885-93.
[http://dx.doi.org/10.1016/S0140-6736(05)67604-0] [PMID: 16310556]

[17] Fatalities and injuries from falls among older adults--United States, 1993-2003 and 2001-2005. MMWR Morb Mortal Wkly Rep 2006; 55(45): 1221-4.
[PMID: 17108890]

[18] Guideline for the prevention of falls in older persons. American Geriatrics Society, British Geriatrics Society, and American Academy of Orthopaedic Surgeons Panel on Falls Prevention. J Am Geriatr

Soc 2001; 49(5): 664-72.
[PMID: 11380764]

[19] Sherrington C, Whitney JC, Lord SR, Herbert RD, Cumming RG, Close JC. Effective exercise for the prevention of falls: a systematic review and meta-analysis. J Am Geriatr Soc 2008; 56(12): 2234-43.
[http://dx.doi.org/10.1111/j.1532-5415.2008.02014.x] [PMID: 19093923]

[20] Robertson MC, Campbell AJ, Gardner MM, Devlin N. Preventing injuries in older people by preventing falls: a meta-analysis of individual-level data. J Am Geriatr Soc 2002; 50(5): 905-11.
[http://dx.doi.org/10.1046/j.1532-5415.2002.50218.x] [PMID: 12028179]

[21] Sawka AM, Boulos P, Beattie K, *et al.* Do hip protectors decrease the risk of hip fracture in institutional and community-dwelling elderly? A systematic review and meta-analysis of randomized controlled trials. Osteoporos Int 2005; 16(12): 1461-74.
[http://dx.doi.org/10.1007/s00198-005-1932-2] [PMID: 15990949]

[22] Duque G, Close JJ, de Jager JP, *et al.* Treatment for osteoporosis in Australian residential aged care facilities: consensus recommendations for fracture prevention. Med J Aust 2010; 193(3): 173-9.
[PMID: 20678047]

[23] Schousboe JT, Nyman JA, Kane RL, Ensrud KE. Cost-effectiveness of alendronate therapy for osteopenic postmenopausal women. Ann Intern Med 2005; 142(9): 734-41.
[http://dx.doi.org/10.7326/0003-4819-142-9-200505030-00008] [PMID: 15867405]

[24] Schousboe JT, Ensrud KE, Nyman JA, Melton LJ III, Kane RL. Universal bone densitometry screening combined with alendronate therapy for those diagnosed with osteoporosis is highly cost-effective for elderly women. J Am Geriatr Soc 2005; 53(10): 1697-704.
[http://dx.doi.org/10.1111/j.1532-5415.2005.53504.x] [PMID: 16181168]

[25] Uihlein AV, Leder BZ. Anabolic therapies for osteoporosis. Endocrinol Metab Clin North Am 2012; 41(3): 507-25.
[http://dx.doi.org/10.1016/j.ecl.2012.05.002] [PMID: 22877427]

[26] Müller D, Pulm J, Gandjour A. Cost-effectiveness of different strategies for selecting and treating individuals at increased risk of osteoporosis or osteopenia: a systematic review. Value Health 2012; 15(2): 284-98.
[http://dx.doi.org/10.1016/j.jval.2011.11.030] [PMID: 22433760]

[27] van den Bergh JP, Bours SP, van Geel TA, Geusens PP. Optimal use of vitamin D when treating osteoporosis. Curr Osteoporos Rep 2011; 9(1): 36-42.
[http://dx.doi.org/10.1007/s11914-010-0041-0] [PMID: 21113692]

[28] Tang BM, Eslick GD, Nowson C, Smith C, Bensoussan A. Use of calcium or calcium in combination with vitamin D supplementation to prevent fractures and bone loss in people aged 50 years and older: a meta-analysis. Lancet 2007; 370(9588): 657-66.
[http://dx.doi.org/10.1016/S0140-6736(07)61342-7] [PMID: 17720017]

[29] Sanders KM, Nowson CA, Kotowicz MA, Briffa K, Devine A, Reid IR. Calcium and bone health: position statement for the Australian and New Zealand Bone and Mineral Society, Osteoporosis Australia and the Endocrine Society of Australia. Med J Aust 2009; 190(6): 316-20.
[PMID: 19296813]

[30] Martin CE, Veysey M, Yates ZR, Lucock MD. Vitamin D: genetics, environment & health. J Food Nutr Disord 2014; 3: 5.
[http://dx.doi.org/10.4172/2324-9323.1000155]

[31] Murad MH, Drake MT, Mullan RJ, *et al.* Clinical review. Comparative effectiveness of drug treatments to prevent fragility fractures: a systematic review and network meta-analysis. J Clin Endocrinol Metab 2012; 97(6): 1871-80.
[http://dx.doi.org/10.1210/jc.2011-3060] [PMID: 22466336]

[32] Khosla S. Update on estrogens and the skeleton. J Clin Endocrinol Metab 2010; 95(8): 3569-77.
[http://dx.doi.org/10.1210/jc.2010-0856] [PMID: 20685883]

[33] Cauley JA, Seeley DG, Ensrud K, Ettinger B, Black D, Cummings SR. Estrogen replacement therapy and fractures in older women. Ann Intern Med 1995; 122(1): 9-16.
[http://dx.doi.org/10.7326/0003-4819-122-1-199501010-00002] [PMID: 7985914]

[34] Manson JE, Chlebowski RT, Stefanick ML, *et al.* Menopausal hormone therapy and health outcomes during the intervention and extended poststopping phases of the Women's Health Initiative randomized trials. JAMA 2013; 310(13): 1353-68.
[http://dx.doi.org/10.1001/jama.2013.278040] [PMID: 24084921]

[35] Marjoribanks J, Farquhar C, Roberts H, Lethaby A. Long term hormone therapy for perimenopausal and postmenopausal women. Cochrane Database Syst Rev 2012; 7: CD004143.
[PMID: 22786488]

[36] Jamal SA, Bauer DC, Ensrud KE, *et al.* Alendronate treatment in women with normal to severely impaired renal function: an analysis of the fracture intervention trial. J Bone Miner Res 2007; 22(4): 503-8.
[http://dx.doi.org/10.1359/jbmr.070112] [PMID: 17243862]

[37] McClung MR, Geusens P, Miller PD, *et al.* Effect of risedronate on the risk of hip fracture in elderly women. N Engl J Med 2001; 344(5): 333-40.
[http://dx.doi.org/10.1056/NEJM200102013440503] [PMID: 11172164]

[38] Boonen S, McClung MR, Eastell R, El-Hajj Fuleihan G, Barton IP, Delmas P. Safety and efficacy of risedronate in reducing fracture risk in osteoporotic women aged 80 and older: implications for the use of antiresorptive agents in the old and oldest old. J Am Geriatr Soc 2004; 52(11): 1832-9.
[http://dx.doi.org/10.1111/j.1532-5415.2004.52506.x] [PMID: 15507059]

[39] Masud T, McClung M, Geusens P. Reducing hip fracture risk with risedronate in elderly women with established osteoporosis. Clin Interv Aging 2009; 4: 445-9.
[http://dx.doi.org/10.2147/CIA.S8200] [PMID: 19966913]

[40] Silverman SL, Schousboe JT, Gold DT. Oral bisphosphonate compliance and persistence: a matter of choice? Osteoporos Int 2011; 22(1): 21-6.
[http://dx.doi.org/10.1007/s00198-010-1274-6] [PMID: 20458571]

[41] Maricic M. The role of zoledronic acid in the management of osteoporosis. Clin Rheumatol 2010; 29(10): 1079-84.
[http://dx.doi.org/10.1007/s10067-010-1486-3] [PMID: 20544246]

[42] Sambrook PN, Roux C, Devogelaer JP, *et al.* Bisphosphonates and glucocorticoid osteoporosis in men:

results of a randomized controlled trial comparing zoledronic acid with risedronate. Bone 2012; 50(1): 289-95.
[http://dx.doi.org/10.1016/j.bone.2011.10.024] [PMID: 22061864]

[43] Lyles KW, Colón-Emeric CS, Magaziner JS, *et al.* Zoledronic acid and clinical fractures and mortality after hip fracture. N Engl J Med 2007; 357(18): 1799-809.
[http://dx.doi.org/10.1056/NEJMoa074941] [PMID: 17878149]

[44] Gamsjaeger S, Buchinger B, Zwettler E, *et al.* Bone material properties in actively bone-forming trabeculae in postmenopausal women with osteoporosis after three years of treatment with once-yearly Zoledronic acid. J Bone Miner Res 2011; 26(1): 12-8.
[http://dx.doi.org/10.1002/jbmr.180] [PMID: 20645415]

[45] Dell RM, Adams AL, Greene DF, *et al.* Incidence of atypical nontraumatic diaphyseal fractures of the femur. J Bone Miner Res 2012; 27(12): 2544-50.
[http://dx.doi.org/10.1002/jbmr.1719] [PMID: 22836783]

[46] Shane E, Burr D, Abrahamsen B, *et al.* Atypical subtrochanteric and diaphyseal femoral fractures: second report of a task force of the American Society for Bone and Mineral Research. J Bone Miner Res 2014; 29(1): 1-23.
[http://dx.doi.org/10.1002/jbmr.1998] [PMID: 23712442]

[47] Reginster JY, Kaufman JM, Goemaere S, *et al.* Maintenance of antifracture efficacy over 10 years with strontium ranelate in postmenopausal osteoporosis. Osteoporos Int 2012; 23(3): 1115-22.
[http://dx.doi.org/10.1007/s00198-011-1847-z] [PMID: 22124575]

[48] Rizzoli R, Reginster JY. Adverse drug reactions to osteoporosis treatments. Expert Rev Clin Pharmacol 2011; 4(5): 593-604.
[http://dx.doi.org/10.1586/ecp.11.42] [PMID: 22220306]

[49] Ettinger B, Black DM, Mitlak BH, *et al.* Reduction of vertebral fracture risk in postmenopausal women with osteoporosis treated with raloxifene: results from a 3-year randomized clinical trial. JAMA 1999; 282(7): 637-45.
[http://dx.doi.org/10.1001/jama.282.7.637] [PMID: 10517716]

[50] Sutton EE, Riche DM. Denosumab, a RANK ligand inhibitor, for postmenopausal women with osteoporosis. Ann Pharmacother 2012; 46(7-8): 1000-9.
[http://dx.doi.org/10.1345/aph.1Q543] [PMID: 22837347]

[51] Cummings SR, San Martin J, McClung MR, *et al.* Denosumab for prevention of fractures in postmenopausal women with osteoporosis. N Engl J Med 2009; 361(8): 756-65.
[http://dx.doi.org/10.1056/NEJMoa0809493] [PMID: 19671655]

[52] Watts NB, Roux C, Modlin JF, *et al.* Infections in postmenopausal women with osteoporosis treated with denosumab or placebo: coincidence or causal association? Osteoporos Int 2012; 23(1): 327-37.
[http://dx.doi.org/10.1007/s00198-011-1755-2] [PMID: 21892677]

[53] Paparodis R, Buehring B, Pelley EM, Binkley N. A case of an unusual subtrochanteric fracture in a patient receiving denosumab. Endocr Pract 2013; 19(3): e64-8.
[http://dx.doi.org/10.4158/EP12367.CR] [PMID: 23337161]

[54] Khow KS, Yong TY. Atypical femoral fracture in a patient treated with denosumab. J Bone Miner

Metab 2015; 33(3): 355-8.
[http://dx.doi.org/10.1007/s00774-014-0606-6] [PMID: 24996528]

[55] Boonen S, Black DM, Colón-Emeric CS, *et al.* Efficacy and safety of a once-yearly intravenous zoledronic acid 5 mg for fracture prevention in elderly postmenopausal women with osteoporosis aged 75 and older. J Am Geriatr Soc 2010; 58(2): 292-9.
[http://dx.doi.org/10.1111/j.1532-5415.2009.02673.x] [PMID: 20070415]

[56] Seeman E, Vellas B, Benhamou C, *et al.* Strontium ranelate reduces the risk of vertebral and nonvertebral fractures in women eighty years of age and older. J Bone Miner Res 2006; 21(7): 1113-20.
[http://dx.doi.org/10.1359/jbmr.060404] [PMID: 16813532]

[57] Boonen S, Adachi JD, Man Z, *et al.* Treatment with denosumab reduces the incidence of new vertebral and hip fractures in postmenopausal women at high risk. J Clin Endocrinol Metab 2011; 96(6): 1727-36.
[http://dx.doi.org/10.1210/jc.2010-2784] [PMID: 21411557]

[58] Neer RM, Arnaud CD, Zanchetta JR, *et al.* Effect of parathyroid hormone (1-34) on fractures and bone mineral density in postmenopausal women with osteoporosis. N Engl J Med 2001; 344(19): 1434-41.
[http://dx.doi.org/10.1056/NEJM200105103441904] [PMID: 11346808]

[59] Boonen S, Marin F, Mellstrom D, *et al.* Safety and efficacy of teriparatide in elderly women with established osteoporosis: bone anabolic therapy from a geriatric perspective. J Am Geriatr Soc 2006; 54(5): 782-9.
[http://dx.doi.org/10.1111/j.1532-5415.2006.00695.x] [PMID: 16696744]

[60] Yu S, Burge RT, Foster SA, Gelwicks S, Meadows ES. The impact of teriparatide adherence and persistence on fracture outcomes. Osteoporos Int 2012; 23(3): 1103-13.
[http://dx.doi.org/10.1007/s00198-011-1843-3] [PMID: 22159748]

[61] Ng KW. Potential role of odanacatib in the treatment of osteoporosis. Clin Interv Aging 2012; 7: 235-47.
[http://dx.doi.org/10.2147/CIA.S26729] [PMID: 22866001]

[62] Bonnick S, De Villiers T, Odio A, *et al.* Effects of odanacatib on BMD and safety in the treatment of osteoporosis in postmenopausal women previously treated with alendronate: a randomized placebo-controlled trial. J Clin Endocrinol Metab 2013; 98(12): 4727-35.
[http://dx.doi.org/10.1210/jc.2013-2020] [PMID: 24064689]

[63] Langdahl B, Binkley N, Bone H, *et al.* Odanacatib in the treatment of postmenopausal women with low bone mineral density: five years of continued therapy in a phase 2 study. J Bone Miner Res 2012; 27(11): 2251-8.
[http://dx.doi.org/10.1002/jbmr.1695] [PMID: 22777865]

[64] Stoch SA, Zajic S, Stone JA, *et al.* Odanacatib, a selective cathepsin K inhibitor to treat osteoporosis: safety, tolerability, pharmacokinetics and pharmacodynamics--results from single oral dose studies in healthy volunteers. Br J Clin Pharmacol 2013; 75(5): 1240-54.
[http://dx.doi.org/10.1111/j.1365-2125.2012.04471.x] [PMID: 23013236]

[65] Lewiecki EM. Sclerostin monoclonal antibody therapy with AMG 785: a potential treatment for osteoporosis. Expert Opin Biol Ther 2011; 11(1): 117-27.

[http://dx.doi.org/10.1517/14712598.2011.540565] [PMID: 21114421]

[66] McClung MR, Grauer A, Boonen S, *et al.* Romosozumab in postmenopausal women with low bone mineral density. N Engl J Med 2014; 370(5): 412-20.
[http://dx.doi.org/10.1056/NEJMoa1305224] [PMID: 24382002]

[67] Cumming RG. Nursing home residence and risk of hip fracture. Am J Epidemiol 1996; 143(12): 1191-4.
[http://dx.doi.org/10.1093/oxfordjournals.aje.a008706] [PMID: 8651217]

[68] Albaum JM, Youn S, Levesque LE, Gershon AS, Cadarette SM. Osteoporosis management among chronic glucocorticoid users: a systematic review. J Popul Ther Clin Pharmacol 2014; 21(3): e486-504.
[PMID: 25527817]

[69] Liu SK, Munson JC, Bell JE, *et al.* Quality of osteoporosis care of older Medicare recipients with fragility fractures: 2006 to 2010. J Am Geriatr Soc 2013; 61(11): 1855-62.
[http://dx.doi.org/10.1111/jgs.12507] [PMID: 24219186]

[70] Feldstein AC, Nichols GA, Elmer PJ, Smith DH, Aickin M, Herson M. Older women with fractures: patients falling through the cracks of guideline-recommended osteoporosis screening and treatment. J Bone Joint Surg Am 2003; 85-A(12): 2294-302.
[PMID: 14668497]

CHAPTER 11

Keep the Kidneys Functioning Till the End: Chronic Kidney Disease in the Older Population

Danielle Wu[1], Tuck Yean Yong[2,*]

[1] *Department of Nephrology, Mackay Base Hospital, Mackay, Queensland, Australia*

[2] *Internal Medicine, Flinders Private Hospital, Flinders Drive, Bedford Park, South Australia 5042, Australia.*

Abstract: With population ageing and increasing life expectancy, the prevalence of chronic kidney disease (CKD) is rising. In addition to its associated cardiovascular risk, CKD in older people have increased prevalence of geriatric syndromes such as cognitive and functional decline, leading to frailty and disability. Clinical trials evaluating treatment for CKD have usually excluded patients older than 70 years, making it difficult to translate current therapeutic recommendation to the older population. Available evidence suggests that patients over 75 years of age with CKD in the presence of multiple comorbidities have greatly reduced life expectancy and quality of life, even if they choose to have renal replacement therapy. Therefore offering a conservative approach to management supported by palliative care is a more reasonable option for some patients. Kidney transplantation can lead to better life expectancy and quality of life in older people if selected carefully. There is a need for the inclusion of older people in future CKD trials so that evidence-based therapies can be offered to this group.

Keywords: Albuminuria, Creatinine, Chronic kidney disease, Dialysis, End-stage kidney disease, Geriatric syndromes, Glomerular filtration rate, Kidney transplantation, Palliative care, Renal replacement therapy.

* **Correspondence author Tuck Yean Yong:** Internal Medicine, Flinders Private Hospital, Flinders Drive, Bedford Park, South Australia 5042, Australia; Tel: +61 8 8241 2121; Fax: +61 8 8240 0879; E-mail: tyyong@hotmail.com.

INTRODUCTION

The proportion of older people (aged >65 years) is steadily increasing worldwide, with rapid growth seen in low and middle-income countries. This demographic change has important implications for health conditions such as chronic kidney disease (CKD), for which the prevalence increases with age.

It is well recognised that estimated glomerular filtration rate (eGFR) declines with increasing age [1]. Relative increases in the prevalence of CKD with age have been reported in the U.S., Canada, China, U.K. and European countries [2]. Furthermore the incidence of dialysis-dependent kidney disease has steadily increased among older people. For example, in the U.S., a 57% age-adjusted increase in the number of octogenarians and nonagenarians starting dialysis was observed between 1996 and 2003 [3].

CHANGES IN THE KIDNEYS WITH INCREASING AGE

Kidney function declines as a normal part of ageing and some of the causes were shown in (Table **1**) [4]. Renal mass decreases with age, secondary to a reduction in the number of glomeruli [1]. It used to be thought that GFR inevitably declined with age, but longitudinal studies now suggest that in about one-third of patients, there is no significant decrease in renal function, even up to the age of 89 years [5, 6]. However, co-morbidities which are prevalent in older people, such as hypertension, cardiovascular disease, and diabetes mellitus, can significantly impact kidney function [7]. The underlying causes of renal failure may not be immediately apparent in some cases because the definitive diagnostic test, renal biopsy, sometimes carries greater risks than benefits in the older population.

Table 1. Kidney changes with increasing age.

1. Decreased size by 20–30% by the age of 70 years
2. Decline in length, number, and thickness of renal tubules
3. Interstitial tissue and tubular diverticula of renal tubules are increased
4. Decrease in renal blood flow by approximately 10% per decade after the age of 20 years
5. Glomerular filtration rate decreases about 10 mL/min per decade
6. Free water absorption decreases by about 5% per decade after the age of 50 years
7. Decrease in effective renal plasma flow is proportionally greater than glomerular filtration rate
8. Accelerated decline in kidney function in the presence of conditions such as hypertension, atherosclerosis, and heart failure

ASSESSING KIDNEY FUNCTION IN OLDER PEOPLE

The Kidney Disease Improving Global Outcomes (KDIGO) published in 2013 did not provide specific recommendations on the early identification and management of CKD in older people [8]. In fact, the current classification may overestimate the prevalence of CKD in the older population [9]. Within the new classification system, age-related cut-off points for the diagnosis of CKD are no longer recommended [10]. This change was based on evidence that reduced eGFR and albuminuria predicted End-Stage Kidney Disease (ESKD) onset and mortality, irrespective of age [11].

Creatinine is not a sensitive marker of kidney function because it can be affected by muscle mass, diet and renal tubular secretion [12]. As a result measurement and reporting of kidney function has evolved from using serum creatinine to complex formulae such as the Cockcroft-Gault [13], Modification of Diet in Renal Disease (MDRD) [14] and Chronic Kidney Disease Epidemiology Collaboration (CKD-EPI) equations [15]. KDIGO currently uses the CKD-EPI formula because it is considered to be more accurate [8]. However it remains unclear how accurate these formulae are in older people and one study have found these equations may misclassify CKD by one stage [16]. To our knowledge, frailty status has not been explicitly considered in validation studies of equations estimatingGFR. However, since sarcopenia is a core feature of the frailty phenotype [17], GFR estimated from plasma creatinine may overestimate the true GFR for older people who are frail.

All creatinine-based equations for estimating eGFR contain an age variable. As age is a strong factor predisposing to all-cause mortality and cardiovascular morbidity and mortality, it can confound the observed relationship between eGFR and these outcomes. Measuring urine albumin excretion might help clarify which older person truly has CKD and is at increased risk for disease-related adverse events [18].

BURDEN OF CKD IN OLDER PEOPLE

In the UK, the prevalence of CKD in people ≥75 years old is 56.1% for eGFR <60, 17.7% for eGFR <45 mL/min/1.73 m^2 and 2.7% for eGFR <30 mL/min/1.73

m^2 [19]. In the NHANES 1999-2004, the prevalence of CKD was 46.8% in people ≥70 years old compared to 6.7% among those aged 40-59 years [15].

In residential aged care facilities, the prevalence of CKD is higher but it tends to be less recognised. In a cross-sectional study of 82 nursing homes across the US, CKD (eGFR <60) was prevalent in about 50% of residents [20]. Of those residents with CKD, 47.6% were in stage 3A (eGFR 45-59 mL/min/1.73 m^2), 39.3% in stage 3B (eGFR 30-44 mL/min/1.73 m^2) and 13.2% in stage 4 or 5 (eGFR <30 mL/min/1.73 m^2). The mean number of comorbidities in this cohort was 5.3. Approximately 57% of those without CKD had five or more comorbidities compared to 87% of those with stage 4 or 5 CKD. A similar study in the UK reported the prevalence of CKD (eGFR <60 mL/min/1.73 m^2) was 82% among 250 residents [21].

It is well documented that CKD is associated with adverse outcomes such as cardiovascular events and mortality which is attributable to a decline in kidney function [22]. In older people, CKD is often associated with additional complications such as frailty, cognitive impairment and decline in physical function.

CKD AND GERIATRIC SYNDROMES

An association between frailty and renal impairment has been observed in several studies. The prevalence of the frailty phenotype is estimated to be 15% in older people with any degree of chronic kidney impairment [7], increasing to 21% among those with stage 3 or higher CKD [23] and 73% at dialysis initiation [24]. Frailty is associated with increased mortality in older people with CKD, even after adjustment for chronological age and comorbidities [25]. However, whether frailty is a cause or consequence of renal impairment has yet to be established.

In older people, CKD is associated with increased prevalence of cognitive decline. In the Intervention Project on Cerebrovascular Diseases and Dementia in the Community of Ebersberg (INVADE) study, involving 3679 participants whose baseline kidney function are categorised into normal, mild and moderate-to-severe dysfunction (eGFR ≥60, 45-59 and <45 mL/min/1.73 m^2, respectively), new cognitive impairment were reported at a rate of 5.8%, 9.9% and 21.5%, respectively, after two years of follow-up [26]. In a Taiwanese study of 37,049 newly diagnosed patients with CKD and 74,098 non-CKD subjects matched for age and gender, the incidence of dementia is significantly higher in the CKD cohort (9.30 *vs.* 5.55 per 1,000 person-years) after adjusting for age, gender, comorbidities and medications [27].

In a two-year study period, older community-dwelling people with eGFR <60 mL/min/1.73 m^2 were associated independently with decline in basic and instrumental activities of daily living [28]. More severe kidney impairment (eGFR <45 mL/min/1.73 m^2) was associated with lower ability to perform activities of daily living. In the setting of CKD, the decline in physical function will eventually lead to disability which is proportional in severity to the degree of renal dysfunction. The association between CKD and functional deterioration is likely to involve multiple factors. Severity of CKD may also reflect severity of underlying conditions such as cardiovascular diseases, hypertension and diabetes. Therefore, a reduced eGFR may be a marker for overall comorbidity burden leading to functional decline rather than a direct single aetiological factor.

In most of the patients with CKD, hip fracture is an injury that can result from a fall. CKD patients are at an increased risk of falls [29 - 31], and it appears to be an important contributor to the increased hip fracture risk. CKD can lead to muscle wasting [32] and limitation of joint motion [33] which predisposes people with the disorder to falls. Furthermore low vitamin D level is one of causes of muscle wasting in CKD [34]. The increased risk of fracture is also due in part to Chronic Kidney Disease-Mineral and Bone Disorder (CKD-MBD). The increased risk of falls is one of the major contributors to elevated hip fracture risk among CKD patients.

MANAGEMENT OF CKD IN OLDER AGE

In general, the management approach to CKD should involve prevention, early diagnosis, slow progression, treatment and reduction of complications associated with low GFR, cardiovascular diseases, initiation of renal replacement therapy (RRT) when appropriate and preservation of quality of life. An individualized approach with a focus on patients' goals is important in older people with CKD.

Goals of therapy will depend on patients' overall health status and their choices. For patients choosing or suitable for active care, aims should focus on cardiovascular risk reduction, management of CKD-associated complications, careful kidney function monitoring, and RRT initiation when appropriate. Elderly patients who are potentially renal transplant recipients need to have relevant pre-renal transplant workup early with a focus to identify possible donors, rule out significant cardiac risk factors, exclude active malignancy, identify adequate social/psychological support, and have careful review by renal transplant specialists to determine their suitability. For patients who choose supportive care or when this option is more realistic, enhancing quality of life becomes a priority and symptom control should be the main focus of management. Involvement of chronic renal failure specialty nurses and/or palliative care team for ongoing education and community support could also be considered when appropriate.

CKD PREVENTION

Lifestyle modifications including weight reduction for those with obesity, regular exercise, healthy diet, and smoking cessation are cornerstones for preventing CKD. These measures are also often beneficial for the management of cardiovascular diseases, hypertension and diabetes, which are major contributors to the development of CKD. Specific dietary measures such as high cereal fibres, long-chain omega-3 fatty acids and fish intake have been found to reduce the incidence and progression of CKD [35, 36].

Reduced GFR is associated with changes in pharmacokinetics and pharmacodynamics of many drugs, leading to an increased risk of adverse effects including nephrotoxicity if the dose is not adjusted appropriately. Many commonly used drugs and procedures can potentially cause acute kidney injury (AKI) and patients with reduced GFR have an increased risk of drug-induced injury [37]. Non-steroidal anti-inflammatory drugs, aminoglycoside antibiotics and iodinated contrasts should be avoided if possible.

CKD is recognised to be a potential risk factor for prescription errors leading to nephrotoxicity [38]. Furthermore, AKI is a frequent complication of these errors and can potentially accelerate progression of CKD [39, 40]. Therefore, regular medication reviews are important to avoid nephrotoxins, ensure appropriate dosing and minimize polypharmacy.

SLOWING THE RATE OF CKD PROGRESSION

Regardless of age, patients with advanced CKD can be managed appropriately to slow the loss of kidney function and better control metabolic consequences. Rate of progression of CKD varies with underlying disease and the presence or absence of albuminuria. Angiotensin-converting enzyme inhibitors and angiotensin receptor blockers are useful in reducing albuminuria and slowing the decline in GFR [8]. However, these medications need to be used with caution in the elderly patients approaching ESKD, especially in those prone to have hyperkalaemia with concurrent use of potassium-sparing diuretics or in patients with reduced urine output to avoid life-threatening hyperkalaemia and further reduction of eGFR.

MANAGEMENT OF CKD COMPLICATIONS

Progressive decline in kidney function is associated with sodium and water retention, metabolic and hormonal changes resulting in increased prevalence of hypertension, anaemia, metabolic acidosis and renal bone disease [41].

The ideal level of blood pressure control and selection of antihypertensive drugs to reduce the risk of cardiovascular diseases are still uncertain. Guidelines suggest a lower than usual target for blood pressure control (<130/80 mmHg) but no adequately powered randomised trials of participants with CKD have been done to prove this hypothesis [8]. Furthermore current guidelines published by the Kidney Disease Improving Global Outcomes (KDIGO) group provides minimal recommendations targeting the care of older people.

Anaemia in CKD is caused by decreased production of erythropoietin, lack of responsiveness of erythropoietin in the bone marrow, increased hepcidin production by the liver and decreased iron availability for erythropoiesis [42]. Like the younger population, the recommendation is to correct the anaemia by targeting haemoglobin of 11-12 g/dL [43]. Iron supplementation should be given to patients with low plasma ferritin. Treatment with erythrocyte-stimulating agents (ESA) increases haemoglobin, reduces the need for transfusions and improves exercise capacity and quality of life [44, 45].

CKD-MBD are characterised by changes in concentrations of serum calcium, phosphate, 1,25-dihydrocholecalciferol and parathyroid hormone; alteration in bone morphology and vascular calcifications [46]. Secondary hyperparathyroidism can be treated with exogenous 1,25-dihydrocholecalciferol and vitamin D analogues, and calcimimetics. Although these measures can prevent osteitis fibrosa cystica, they do not reduce the incidence of fractures which is a significant concern in older people [47].

DIALYSIS

With the increasing prevalence of CKD and ESKD among older people, the use of RRT by this group is expected to increase [48]. The Australian Institute of Health and Welfare data showed that the number of older people who die with ESKD is similar to those who are accepted for dialysis in 2003-2007 [49].

In developed countries, management approach for older people with ESKD is shifting from conservative management to initiation of dialysis [50]. Observational studies of older people with ESKD have found that initiation of dialysis was not associated with improved survival for those aged >75 years with two or more comorbidities [3, 51, 52].

Available evidence suggests dialysis is an appropriate treatment option for well-informed older people with ESKD and good baseline quality of life. However the poor outcomes experienced by those with multiple comorbidities or lower functional status at baseline clearly demonstrate that dialysis does not always lead to the desired results for older people with ESKD [3]. Therefore sound clinical judgement and careful communications with older patients and their family are required to ensure the appropriate patients are initiated on dialysis.

It is uncertain how applicable the desired clinical targets and quality of care are for older people with ESKD because clinical trials have often excluded people over the age of 75 years. Future researches are needed to address the outcomes of placing older people greater than 75 years on dialysis.

In Australia, withdrawal of dialysis is a common cause of death for patients aged

65 and over placed on dialysis [53]. Once decision to withdraw dialysis is confirmed, symptom control and palliative care becomes the main focus of management [54].

KIDNEY TRANSPLANTATION

Recipient age is an important consideration in the allocation of deceased donor kidneys. In general, advanced age *per se* is not an absolute contraindication for kidney transplantation. Kidney transplantation may provide older people with good long-term graft survival and improved quality of life but they have a higher risk of opportunistic infections, cardiovascular diseases and cancer than their younger counterparts [55]. Kidney transplantation has been found to reduce mortality among patients of all ages [56].

In view of organ shortage, use of expanded criteria deceased donors [57, 58], and more liberal use of older living donors [59] has been found to reduce mortality among older people with kidney failure, when compared with similar patients who remain on the transplant waiting list. These two strategies are particularly appealing to overcome organ shortage and to meet the needs for kidney transplantation among older ESKD patients which is increasing in prevalence. However because the transplant surgery increases the risk of short-term death, the long-term mortality benefits associated with kidney transplantation (regardless of donor type) are limited to those with reasonable baseline life expectancy [60].

FUTURE RESEARCH

Many therapeutic trials for CKD have excluded older people [61] and inclusion of this age group in future trials will improve the ability to translate research into practice. There is also a lack of guidelines on how to manage many complex comorbidities that are associated with CKD which may lead to competing therapeutic priorities. More studies are needed to evaluate the best approach to optimising quality of life and manage symptoms in older people with CKD or ESKD including those who have chosen to be managed conservatively. More accurate tools are needed to identify the subset of patients who can expect a reasonable life expectancy and quality of life if they choose to have dialysis.

CONCLUSION

Population ageing means that older people are accounting for an increasing proportion of patients with or at risk for CKD and ESKD. Regardless of age, with appropriate management, patients with CKD may benefit from slowing the rate of kidney function decline, better control of metabolic consequences such as metabolic acidosis, renal anaemia, hyperkalaemia, hypocalcaemia, hyperphosphataemia, CKD-MBD, uraemic symptoms and risk of cardiovascular events. Older people with ESKD should be engaged in a more informed decision-making about RRT modality if appropriate.

CONFLICT OF INTEREST

The author confirms that author has no conflict of interest to declare for this publication.

ACKNOWLEDGEMENTS

Declared none.

KEY POINTS

- Prevalence of chronic kidney disease in older people is rising due to population ageing and increase in life expectancy.
- Cardiovascular mortality is the major outcome in a large proportion of older people with chronic kidney disease.
- Older people with chronic kidney disease are at increased risk of developing geriatric syndromes such as cognitive decline, frailty and physical decline.
- Management of chronic kidney disease in the older population should take into consideration realistic outcomes that can be achieved in this age group.
- A holistic approach in management should be adopted in older patients with chronic kidney disease to achieve an appropriate quality of life.

REFERENCES

[1] Glassock RJ, Rule AD. The implications of anatomical and functional changes of the aging kidney: with an emphasis on the glomeruli. Kidney Int 2012; 82(3): 270-7. [http://dx.doi.org/10.1038/ki.2012.65] [PMID: 22437416]

[2] Tonelli M, Riella MC. Chronic kidney disease and the aging population. Kidney Int 2014; 85(3): 487-91.
[http://dx.doi.org/10.1038/ki.2013.467] [PMID: 24336028]

[3] Kurella M, Covinsky KE, Collins AJ, Chertow GM. Octogenarians and nonagenarians starting dialysis in the United States. Ann Intern Med 2007; 146(3): 177-83.
[http://dx.doi.org/10.7326/0003-4819-146-3-200702060-00006] [PMID: 17283348]

[4] Zhou XJ, Rakheja D, Yu X, Saxena R, Vaziri ND, Silva FG. The aging kidney. Kidney Int 2008; 74(6): 710-20.
[http://dx.doi.org/10.1038/ki.2008.319] [PMID: 18614996]

[5] Lindeman RD, Tobin J, Shock NW. Longitudinal studies on the rate of decline in renal function with age. J Am Geriatr Soc 1985; 33(4): 278-85.
[http://dx.doi.org/10.1111/j.1532-5415.1985.tb07117.x] [PMID: 3989190]

[6] Fehrman-Ekholm I, Skeppholm L. Renal function in the elderly (>70 years old) measured by means of iohexol clearance, serum creatinine, serum urea and estimated clearance. Scand J Urol Nephrol 2004; 38(1): 73-7.
[http://dx.doi.org/10.1080/00365590310015750] [PMID: 15204431]

[7] Shlipak MG, Stehman-Breen C, Fried LF, *et al.* The presence of frailty in elderly persons with chronic renal insufficiency. Am J Kidney Dis 2004; 43(5): 861-7.
[http://dx.doi.org/10.1053/j.ajkd.2003.12.049] [PMID: 15112177]

[8] Chapter 3: Management of progression and complications of CKD. Kidney Int Suppl (2011) 2013; 3(1): 73-90.
[http://dx.doi.org/10.1038/kisup.2012.66] [PMID: 25598999]

[9] Dousdampanis P, Trigka K, Fourtounas C. Diagnosis and management of chronic kidney disease in the elderly: a field of ongoing debate. Aging Dis 2012; 3(5): 360-72.
[PMID: 23185717]

[10] Johnson DW, Jones GR, Mathew TH, *et al.* Chronic kidney disease and measurement of albuminuria or proteinuria: a position statement. Med J Aust 2012; 197(4): 224-5.
[http://dx.doi.org/10.5694/mja11.11468] [PMID: 22900872]

[11] Hallan SI, Matsushita K, Sang Y, *et al.* Age and association of kidney measures with mortality and end-stage renal disease. JAMA 2012; 308(22): 2349-60.
[http://dx.doi.org/10.1001/jama.2012.16817] [PMID: 23111824]

[12] Epstein M. Aging and the kidney. J Am Soc Nephrol 1996; 7(8): 1106-22.
[PMID: 8866401]

[13] Cockcroft DW, Gault MH. Prediction of creatinine clearance from serum creatinine. Nephron 1976; 16(1): 31-41.
[http://dx.doi.org/10.1159/000180580] [PMID: 1244564]

[14] Levey AS, Bosch JP, Lewis JB, Greene T, Rogers N, Roth D. A more accurate method to estimate glomerular filtration rate from serum creatinine: a new prediction equation. Ann Intern Med 1999; 130(6): 461-70.
[http://dx.doi.org/10.7326/0003-4819-130-6-199903160-00002] [PMID: 10075613]

[15] Levey AS, Stevens LA, Schmid CH, *et al.* A new equation to estimate glomerular filtration rate. Ann Intern Med 2009; 150(9): 604-12.
[http://dx.doi.org/10.7326/0003-4819-150-9-200905050-00006] [PMID: 19414839]

[16] Drenth-van Maanen AC, Jansen PA, Proost JH, *et al.* Renal function assessment in older adults. Br J Clin Pharmacol 2013; 76(4): 616-23.
[PMID: 23802656]

[17] Fried LP, Tangen CM, Walston J, *et al.* Frailty in older adults: evidence for a phenotype. J Gerontol A Biol Sci Med Sci 2001; 56(3): M146-56.
[http://dx.doi.org/10.1093/gerona/56.3.M146] [PMID: 11253156]

[18] Muntner P, Bowling CB, Gao L, *et al.* Age-specific association of reduced estimated glomerular filtration rate and albuminuria with all-cause mortality. Clin J Am Soc Nephrol 2011; 6(9): 2200-7.
[http://dx.doi.org/10.2215/CJN.02030311] [PMID: 21737849]

[19] Roderick PJ, Atkins RJ, Smeeth L, *et al.* Detecting chronic kidney disease in older people; what are the implications? Age Ageing 2008; 37(2): 179-86.
[http://dx.doi.org/10.1093/ageing/afm180] [PMID: 18083723]

[20] McClellan WM, Resnick B, Lei L, *et al.* Prevalence and severity of chronic kidney disease and anemia in the nursing home population. J Am Med Dir Assoc 2010; 11(1): 33-41.
[http://dx.doi.org/10.1016/j.jamda.2009.07.003] [PMID: 20129213]

[21] Carter JL, O'Riordan SE, Eaglestone GL, Delaney MP, Lamb EJ. Chronic kidney disease prevalence in a UK residential care home population. Nephrol Dial Transplant 2008; 23(4): 1257-64.
[http://dx.doi.org/10.1093/ndt/gfm792] [PMID: 18029370]

[22] Go AS, Chertow GM, Fan D, McCulloch CE, Hsu CY. Chronic kidney disease and the risks of death, cardiovascular events, and hospitalization. N Engl J Med 2004; 351(13): 1296-305.
[http://dx.doi.org/10.1056/NEJMoa041031] [PMID: 15385656]

[23] Wilhelm-Leen ER, Hall YN. Chertow GM. Frailty and chronic kidney disease: the Third National Health and Nutrition Evaluation Survey. Am J Med 2009; 122: 664-671e2.

[24] Bao Y, Dalrymple L, Chertow GM, Kaysen GA, Johansen KL. Frailty, dialysis initiation, and mortality in end-stage renal disease. Arch Intern Med 2012; 172(14): 1071-7.
[http://dx.doi.org/10.1001/archinternmed.2012.3020] [PMID: 22733312]

[25] Johansen KL, Chertow GM, Jin C, Kutner NG. Significance of frailty among dialysis patients. J Am Soc Nephrol 2007; 18(11): 2960-7.
[http://dx.doi.org/10.1681/ASN.2007020221] [PMID: 17942958]

[26] Etgen T, Sander D, Chonchol M, *et al.* Chronic kidney disease is associated with incident cognitive impairment in the elderly: the INVADE study. Nephrol Dial Transplant 2009; 24(10): 3144-50.
[http://dx.doi.org/10.1093/ndt/gfp230] [PMID: 19461010]

[27] Cheng KC, Chen YL, Lai SW, Mou CH, Tsai PY, Sung FC. Patients with chronic kidney disease are at an elevated risk of dementia: a population-based cohort study in Taiwan. BMC Nephrol 2012; 13: 129.
[http://dx.doi.org/10.1186/1471-2369-13-129] [PMID: 23020192]

[28] Bowling CB, Sawyer P, Campbell RC, Ahmed A, Allman RM. Impact of chronic kidney disease on activities of daily living in community-dwelling older adults. J Gerontol A Biol Sci Med Sci 2011; 66(6): 689-94.
[http://dx.doi.org/10.1093/gerona/glr043] [PMID: 21459762]

[29] Cook WL, Tomlinson G, Donaldson M, *et al.* Falls and fall-related injuries in older dialysis patients. Clin J Am Soc Nephrol 2006; 1(6): 1197-204.
[http://dx.doi.org/10.2215/CJN.01650506] [PMID: 17699348]

[30] Desmet C, Beguin C, Swine C, Jadoul M. Falls in hemodialysis patients: prospective study of incidence, risk factors, and complications. Am J Kidney Dis 2005; 45(1): 148-53.
[http://dx.doi.org/10.1053/j.ajkd.2004.09.027] [PMID: 15696454]

[31] Rossier A, Pruijm M, Hannane D, Burnier M, Teta D. Incidence, complications and risk factors for severe falls in patients on maintenance haemodialysis. Nephrol Dial Transplant 2012; 27(1): 352-7.
[http://dx.doi.org/10.1093/ndt/gfr326] [PMID: 21652549]

[32] Workeneh BT, Mitch WE. Review of muscle wasting associated with chronic kidney disease. Am J Clin Nutr 2010; 91(4): 1128S-32S.
[http://dx.doi.org/10.3945/ajcn.2010.28608B] [PMID: 20181807]

[33] Kazama JJ, Yamamoto S, Takahashi N, *et al.* Abeta-2M-amyloidosis and related bone diseases. J Bone Miner Metab 2006; 24(2): 182-4.
[http://dx.doi.org/10.1007/s00774-005-0669-5] [PMID: 16502130]

[34] Boudville N, Inderjeeth C, Elder GJ, Glendenning P. Association between 25-hydroxyvitamin D, somatic muscle weakness and falls risk in end-stage renal failure. Clin Endocrinol (Oxf) 2010; 73(3): 299-304.
[http://dx.doi.org/10.1111/j.1365-2265.2010.03821.x] [PMID: 20507339]

[35] Gopinath B, Harris DC, Flood VM, Burlutsky G, Brand-Miller J, Mitchell P. Carbohydrate nutrition is associated with the 5-year incidence of chronic kidney disease. J Nutr 2011; 141(3): 433-9.
[http://dx.doi.org/10.3945/jn.110.134304] [PMID: 21228263]

[36] Gopinath B, Harris DC, Flood VM, Burlutsky G, Mitchell P. Consumption of long-chain n-3 PUFA, α-linolenic acid and fish is associated with the prevalence of chronic kidney disease. Br J Nutr 2011; 105(9): 1361-8.
[http://dx.doi.org/10.1017/S0007114510005040] [PMID: 21255476]

[37] Hug BL, Witkowski DJ, Sox CM, *et al.* Occurrence of adverse, often preventable, events in community hospitals involving nephrotoxic drugs or those excreted by the kidney. Kidney Int 2009; 76(11): 1192-8.
[http://dx.doi.org/10.1038/ki.2009.353] [PMID: 19759525]

[38] Fink JC, Brown J, Hsu VD, Seliger SL, Walker L, Zhan M. CKD as an underrecognized threat to patient safety. Am J Kidney Dis 2009; 53(4): 681-8.
[http://dx.doi.org/10.1053/j.ajkd.2008.12.016] [PMID: 19246142]

[39] Hsu CY, Ordoñez JD, Chertow GM, Fan D, McCulloch CE, Go AS. The risk of acute renal failure in patients with chronic kidney disease. Kidney Int 2008; 74(1): 101-7.
[http://dx.doi.org/10.1038/ki.2008.107] [PMID: 18385668]

[40] James MT, Hemmelgarn BR, Wiebe N, *et al.* Glomerular filtration rate, proteinuria, and the incidence and consequences of acute kidney injury: a cohort study. Lancet 2010; 376(9758): 2096-103. [http://dx.doi.org/10.1016/S0140-6736(10)61271-8] [PMID: 21094997]

[41] Meyer TW, Hostetter TH. Uremia. N Engl J Med 2007; 357(13): 1316-25. [http://dx.doi.org/10.1056/NEJMra071313] [PMID: 17898101]

[42] Babitt JL, Lin HY. Molecular mechanisms of hepcidin regulation: implications for the anemia of CKD. Am J Kidney Dis 2010; 55(4): 726-41. [http://dx.doi.org/10.1053/j.ajkd.2009.12.030] [PMID: 20189278]

[43] Locatelli F, Nissenson AR, Barrett BJ, *et al.* Clinical practice guidelines for anemia in chronic kidney disease: problems and solutions. A position statement from Kidney Disease: Improving Global Outcomes (KDIGO). Kidney Int 2008; 74(10): 1237-40. [http://dx.doi.org/10.1038/ki.2008.299] [PMID: 18596731]

[44] Gandra SR, Finkelstein FO, Bennett AV, Lewis EF, Brazg T, Martin ML. Impact of erythropoiesis-stimulating agents on energy and physical function in nondialysis CKD patients with anemia: a systematic review. Am J Kidney Dis 2010; 55(3): 519-34. [http://dx.doi.org/10.1053/j.ajkd.2009.09.019] [PMID: 20031287]

[45] Johansen KL, Finkelstein FO, Revicki DA, Gitlin M, Evans C, Mayne TJ. Systematic review and meta-analysis of exercise tolerance and physical functioning in dialysis patients treated with erythropoiesis-stimulating agents. Am J Kidney Dis 2010; 55(3): 535-48. [http://dx.doi.org/10.1053/j.ajkd.2009.12.018] [PMID: 20133033]

[46] KDIGO clinical practice guideline for the diagnosis, evaluation, prevention, and treatment of Chronic Kidney Disease-Mineral and Bone Disorder (CKD-MBD). Kidney Int Suppl 2009; (113): S1-S130. [PMID: 19644521]

[47] Toussaint ND, Elder GJ, Kerr PG. A rational guide to reducing fracture risk in dialysis patients. Semin Dial 2010; 23(1): 43-54. [http://dx.doi.org/10.1111/j.1525-139X.2009.00650.x] [PMID: 20331818]

[48] Grace B. New patients commencing treatment in 2011. Annual Report. 35th ed. Adelaide, Australia: ANZDATA Registry 2012. Chapter 2

[49] Sparke C, Moon L, Green F, *et al.* Estimating the total incidence of kidney failure in Australia including individuals who are not treated by dialysis or transplantation. Am J Kidney Dis 2013; 61(3): 413-9. [http://dx.doi.org/10.1053/j.ajkd.2012.10.012] [PMID: 23177731]

[50] Thorsteinsdottir B, Montori VM, Prokop LJ, Murad MH. Ageism *vs.* the technical imperative, applying the GRADE framework to the evidence on hemodialysis in very elderly patients. Clin Interv Aging 2013; 8: 797-807. [http://dx.doi.org/10.2147/CIA.S43817] [PMID: 23847412]

[51] Murtagh FE, Marsh JE, Donohoe P, Ekbal NJ, Sheerin NS, Harris FE. Dialysis or not? A comparative survival study of patients over 75 years with chronic kidney disease stage 5. Nephrol Dial Transplant 2007; 22(7): 1955-62. [http://dx.doi.org/10.1093/ndt/gfm153] [PMID: 17412702]

[52] Chandna SM, Da Silva-Gane M, Marshall C, Warwicker P, Greenwood RN, Farrington K. Survival of elderly patients with stage 5 CKD: comparison of conservative management and renal replacement therapy. Nephrol Dial Transplant 2011; 26(5): 1608-14.
[http://dx.doi.org/10.1093/ndt/gfq630] [PMID: 21098012]

[53] McDonald S. Deaths. Annual Report. 35th ed. Adelaide, Australia: ANZDATA Registry 2012. Chapter 3

[54] Douglas C, Murtagh FE, Chambers EJ, Howse M, Ellershaw J. Symptom management for the adult patient dying with advanced chronic kidney disease: a review of the literature and development of evidence-based guidelines by a United Kingdom Expert Consensus Group. Palliat Med 2009; 23(2): 103-10.
[http://dx.doi.org/10.1177/0269216308100247] [PMID: 19273566]

[55] Lenihan CR, Hurley MP, Tan JC. Comorbidities and kidney transplant evaluation in the elderly. Am J Nephrol 2013; 38(3): 204-11.
[http://dx.doi.org/10.1159/000354483] [PMID: 23988670]

[56] Knoll GA. Kidney transplantation in the older adult. Am J Kidney Dis 2013; 61(5): 790-7.
[http://dx.doi.org/10.1053/j.ajkd.2012.08.049] [PMID: 23261121]

[57] Merion RM, Ashby VB, Wolfe RA, *et al.* Deceased-donor characteristics and the survival benefit of kidney transplantation. JAMA 2005; 294(21): 2726-33.
[http://dx.doi.org/10.1001/jama.294.21.2726] [PMID: 16333008]

[58] Cohen B, Smits JM, Haase B, Persijn G, Vanrenterghem Y, Frei U. Expanding the donor pool to increase renal transplantation. Nephrol Dial Transplant 2005; 20(1): 34-41.
[http://dx.doi.org/10.1093/ndt/gfh506] [PMID: 15522904]

[59] Gill J, Bunnapradist S, Danovitch GM, Gjertson D, Gill JS, Cecka M. Outcomes of kidney transplantation from older living donors to older recipients. Am J Kidney Dis 2008; 52(3): 541-52.
[http://dx.doi.org/10.1053/j.ajkd.2008.05.017] [PMID: 18653267]

[60] Gill JS, Tonelli M, Johnson N, Kiberd B, Landsberg D, Pereira BJ. The impact of waiting time and comorbid conditions on the survival benefit of kidney transplantation. Kidney Int 2005; 68(5): 2345-51.
[http://dx.doi.org/10.1111/j.1523-1755.2005.00696.x] [PMID: 16221239]

[61] O'Hare AM, Kaufman JS, Covinsky KE, Landefeld CS, McFarland LV, Larson EB. Current guidelines for using angiotensin-converting enzyme inhibitors and angiotensin II-receptor antagonists in chronic kidney disease: is the evidence base relevant to older adults? Ann Intern Med 2009; 150(10): 717-24.
[http://dx.doi.org/10.7326/0003-4819-150-10-200905190-00010] [PMID: 19451579]

CHAPTER 12

End of Life Care in Older People

Kareeann Sok Fun Khow[1,*], Tuck Yean Yong[2]

[1] *Aged and Extended Care Services, The Queen Elizabeth Hospital and Department of Medicine, University of Adelaide, Adelaide, South Australia, Australia*

[2] *Internal Medicine, Flinders Private Hospital, Flinders Drive, Bedford Park, South Australia 5042, Australia*

Abstract: The end-of-life support older people receive is an important aspect of high quality health and social care, especially for those with chronic diseases. To provide high-quality end-of-life care, it is important to clarify with patients their values and goals in treatment through advanced care planning. Such an approach improves the concordance between expressed preferences for care and delivery of care as well as the satisfaction with care. Available research indicates that majority of older people would like the opportunity to discuss their end-of-life care but there are still barriers to such conversations. End-of-life care of older people with chronic diseases should focus on identifying and treating symptoms. Therefore, in end-of-life care, medications which are not intended for symptom control should be avoided.

Keywords: Advance care planning, Carers, Decision-making, Dying, End-of-life, Palliative care, Quality of life, Resuscitation, Terminally ill, Treatment withdrawal.

INTRODUCTION

Supporting older people towards the end of their lives is an important part of high quality health and social care. People are living longer with a high prevalence of multiple chronic diseases and frailty resulting in a growing population requiring complex support even at the end of their lives.

* **Correspondence author Kareeann Sok Fun Khow:** Aged and Extended Care Services, The Queen Elizabeth Hospital, Woodville Road, Woodville South, South Australia 5011, Australia; Tel: +61 8 8222 6000; Fax: +61 8 8222 8593; E-mail: kareeann.khow@adelaide.edu.au.

Therefore providing end-of-life care for the older population often involves ethically and medically challenging decision-making which requires health professionals to carefully consider patients' multiple comorbidities, their quality of life and their wishes regarding treatments.

In general, end-of-life is characterised by health problems accumulating over a period of weeks to months with irreversible pathophysiological changes which leads inevitably to death. Recognizing this end-of-life phase can be challenging for many health professionals and usually requires repeated evaluations over a period of several days or even weeks. The terminal phase of illness indicates that death is imminent, generally within hours or days. Therefore, end-of-life can be viewed as the broader continuum of the terminally ill state.

For health professionals, providing good quality end-of-life care can be challenging and complex. Even with widespread professional acknowledgment of the importance of palliative care, clinicians are often unaware of patients' wishes regarding end-of-life care, interventions are often inconsistent with patients' preferences, and some patients still die in moderate or severe pain [1, 2]. Technology-filled end-of-life care is often associated with reduced quality of life, lower satisfaction of care and increased anxiety for carers and families [3].

This chapter will look at the attitudes of the public and clinicians to advance care planning discussions in older and frail people. In addition, it will also review general aspects of end-of-life care and the prescription of medications for older people in this setting.

RECOGNISING END-OF-LIFE

For a long time, clinicians have recognized that there are circumstances in which patients can no longer benefit from, or do not wish to continue with the burdens of life-sustaining therapies. With their medical expertise and advocacy for patients, physicians have an important responsibility to share clinical prognoses with their patients and families.

Before any good-quality plans for end-of-life patients can be implemented, it is important to first recognise end-of-life itself. A number of symptoms and signs indicating end of life are shown in Table **1** [4].

Table 1. Signs and symptoms indicative of end-of-life.

1. Dependent for all activities of daily living; requiring assistance of caregivers to survive; urine and faecal incontinence
2. Severe impairment of expressive and receptive communication often limited to single words or nonsense phrases
3. Eating or feeding difficulties; loss of ability to recognise food, self-feed, swallow effectively; refusal to eat and drink with weight loss; persistent inability to eat when fed
4. Loss of ability to walk followed up by inability to stand, problems in maintaining sitting posture and subsequently loss of head and neck control, eventually bed bound
5. Development of contractures because of muscle rigidity and deconditioning
6. Persistent confusion, agitation, withdrawal, lethargy or apathy
7. Recurrent infections
8. Having no recognition of family/friends/everyday objects

Adapted from Recognise End of Life and Care Holistically (REACH) toolkit [4].

THE PUBLIC'S ATTITUDE TO END-OF-LIFE CARE DISCUSSIONS

A number of studies have consistently reported that between 61% and 91% of older people would like to discuss their end-of-life care [5 - 9]. Older people saw the benefits of discussions to include assurance that their wishes would be taken into consideration, the opportunity to address important issues of care before developing cognitive impairment or serious illnesses [6]. However there are also studies indicating some older people preferring to 'live one day at a time' [10] and postpone making plans until they were older or in worse health [11].

Most older people wanted discussions on end-of-life care sooner rather than later [7 - 9, 12]. These participants perceived the risk of 'leaving it too late' and recognized the benefits of early discussions would outweigh any discomfort [8]. However there are studies reporting that some older people would defer such discussions till the onset of a terminal or debilitating illness triggering the need for such plans [11, 13].

ARE END-OF-LIFE CARE DISCUSSIONS BEING HELD?

Studies have found that only 2-29% of frail older people had discussed and made some form of end-of-life care plans with a healthcare professional [12, 14 - 16]. There is also often disparity between conversations that patients have held with their family members and with healthcare professionals about end-of-life care planning [16]. In addition, between 15% and 66% of older people were observed to have end-of-life care plans documented in their medical records [5, 10, 17].

HEALTHCARE PROFESSIONALS' ATTITUDE TO END-OF-LIFE CARE DISCUSSIONS

Most clinicians viewed discussions on end-of-life care to be an important part of their professional responsibility [8, 18]. Many of them viewed such discussions to be important with patients who have severe chronic illness (91%) or terminal illness (97%) but less (64%) for older people regardless of their health status [18].While some clinicians did not find such discussion stressful [18], others have commented on the challenges with discussing end-of-life care with frail older people with multiple comorbidities [19]. There is also considerable diversity in opinion of when to initiate discussions about end-of-life care [7, 8, 19].

BARRIERS TO DISCUSSING END-OF-LIFE CARE

A number of themes emerge in the medical literature about barriers to discussing end-of-life care: (a) families, (b) professional and time limitations, (c) patients' reluctance to discuss, and (d) lack of decision-making capacity by patients.

The most frequently identified barrier to discussions of end-of-life care plans are the families of older people. It has been reported that they were sometimes unwilling to discuss these care plans or to accept that their relative is approaching end of life [20, 21]. Lack of close family and breakdown in family relationships are other obstacles identified [11].

Perceived lack of continuity of care and support from healthcare professionals have been identified as another barrier to discussing end-of-life care plans [11, 18]. Health professionals also reported time constraints to hold these conversations [18, 19].

Older frail people were found sometimes to be unwilling to discuss their end-of-life care or wanting to put off discussions to a time 'if I ever have a terminal illness' [6, 11, 19]. Some patients saw end-of-life care discussions as the responsibility of others, particularly family members [9, 13].

Cognitive impairment and a lack of decision-making capacity were felt to be important barriers to planning [11, 20, 22]. Therefore the onset of cognitive impairment should be used as a prompt to initiate end-of-life care discussions.

ADVANCE CARE PLANNING

Advance care planning (ACP) is a process of identifying and facilitating goals of care with the patient so that symptoms are managed, the dying process is not unnecessarily prolonged and their wishes are communicated in the event they are unable to voice decisions for themselves [23]. The processes in ACP are well described and involve a systematic as well as personalised approach [24]. ACP involves structured iterative conversations about goals, values and preferences for end-of-life care which usually occur over several encounters. Randomised trials have shown that ACP improves concordance between expressed preferences for care and delivery of care, provides greater patient and carer satisfaction with care and reduces conflicts in decision-making [25]. Studies have also shown that ACP decreased use of acute hospital beds as well as more and earlier use of palliative care services [26, 27].

Planning for end-of-life and palliative situations should be incorporated into the medical review of older people with chronic diseases [21]. Management of chronic diseases and associated complications is intended to treat pain, promote comfort, improve quality of life and prevent avoidable hospitalisations [25, 26]. Treatment targets needs to be individualised according to expected survival time, but these targets are not relevant in the terminal stage. This planning should not be viewed as an activity only to be undertaken near to the time of death, but as an opportunity to plan for other events along the path of declining health, such as the need for admission to hospital or treatment of intercurrent infection.

PALLIATIVE CARE FOR OLDER PEOPLE

The major focus of palliative care is to provide relief of suffering through the identification and effective treatment of symptoms. The spectrum of symptoms in older people at the end of life differs from younger people because dementia, delirium, urinary incontinence and falls are more common [28]. In older people with chronic diseases, the prevalence of symptoms is high but these are often not recognized. In a study of community-dwelling people (aged ≥60 years) with heart failure, chronic obstructive pulmonary disease or cancer, 86% reported at least one moderate to severe symptom and 69% had at least two such symptoms [29].

Several validated instruments such as the Edmonton Symptom Assessment Scale (ESAS), the Memorial Symptom Assessment Scale (MSAS) or the Rotterdam Symptom Checklist, can provide useful information regarding the presence and severity of symptoms [30 - 32]. ESAS may be more useful because it is shorter than the other tools and is aimed at recognizing symptoms commonly affecting older people with advanced chronic diseases.

Older people often have cognitive, motor, visual or auditory impairments that have to be taken into consideration when assessing the presence and severity of symptoms. In patients with severe cognitive impairment who are unable to communicate appropriately, pain and other symptoms are often difficult to identify and may manifest as agitation, increased confusion or decreased mobility [33]. Therefore the methods of assessment should be modified accordingly.

In general, the same principles as that in younger people are applied to palliative symptom management in older people. However, differences in pharmacokinetics and side effect profiles of medications in older people need to be considered carefully. Therefore, these factors may affect the selection and dose of medications in the older population.

MEDICATION PRESCRIPTION IN THE END-OF-LIFE STAGE

Medication use in the terminal phase of life is well-defined and evidence-based because its focus is primarily and appropriately on symptom management. However there is no proper guideline for clinicians regarding appropriate medication prescribing for patients in the end-of-life stage [34].

In end-of-life care, defining treatment goals is of utmost importance which will in turn direct the most appropriate medication prescription. This process requires discussion between the clinician and the patient as well as caregivers when necessary. "Life-extending" drugs are usually not appropriate in the end-of-life care. In general, drugs for primary prevention have no place in the treatment of older people at the end-of-life because the time-to-benefit is usually longer than life expectancy [34]. Drugs for secondary prevention also need to be reviewed carefully and should be prescribed only if ongoing benefit is to be expected within a patient's life expectancy. Optimisation of medication use for an older person at the end of life is a dynamic process. Several changes may be required over time before medications can be rationalised effectively. When possible, it is preferable that drug withdrawal is done one at a time so that adverse symptoms after discontinuation can be assessed more specifically and necessary corrective actions taken.

CONCLUSION

Most older people are comfortable about discussing their end-of-life care and many welcome the opportunity to do so. Therefore all healthcare professionals need to be more involved in end-of-life care discussions, assist patients and their carers to express what they see as important goals of care and ensure clinical interventions align with these goals. At the end of life, the focus should be on symptom management and medication use need to be optimised. Validated instruments may assist in determining the presence and severity of symptoms.

CONFLICT OF INTEREST

The author confirms that author has no conflict of interest to declare for this publication.

ACKNOWLEDGEMENTS

Declared none.

KEY POINTS

- Technology-driven end-of-life care in older people is often associated with poorer quality of life and lower satisfaction with care.
- Advanced care planning is a process of identifying and planning what patients consider important for a dignified death.
- Majority of older people would like the opportunity to discuss their end-of-life care but most healthcare professionals felt limited by time pressures and the

absence of precipitating event to initiate such discussions.

- Advanced care planning improves concordance between expressed preferences for care and delivered care as well as provides better satisfaction of care for older patients and their caregivers.

REFERENCES

[1] A controlled trial to improve care for seriously ill hospitalized patients. The study to understand prognoses and preferences for outcomes and risks of treatments (SUPPORT). JAMA 1995; 274(20): 1591-8.
[http://dx.doi.org/10.1001/jama.1995.03530200027032] [PMID: 7474243]

[2] Hofmann JC, Wenger NS, Davis RB, *et al.* Patient preferences for communication with physicians about end-of-life decisions. Ann Intern Med 1997; 127(1): 1-12.
[http://dx.doi.org/10.7326/0003-4819-127-1-199707010-00001] [PMID: 9214246]

[3] Wright AA, Zhang B, Ray A, *et al.* Associations between end-of-life discussions, patient mental health, medical care near death, and caregiver bereavement adjustment. JAMA 2008; 300(14): 1665-73.
[http://dx.doi.org/10.1001/jama.300.14.1665] [PMID: 18840840]

[4] Potter JM, Fernando R, Humpel N. Development and evaluation of the REACH (recognise end of life and care holistically) out in dementia toolkit. Australas J Ageing 2013; 32(4): 241-6.
[http://dx.doi.org/10.1111/ajag.12062] [PMID: 24251787]

[5] Stelter KL, Elliott BA, Bruno CA. Living will completion in older adults. Arch Intern Med 1992; 152(5): 954-9.
[http://dx.doi.org/10.1001/archinte.1992.00400170044008] [PMID: 1580721]

[6] Morrison RS, Morrison EW, Glickman DF. Physician reluctance to discuss advance directives. An empiric investigation of potential barriers. Arch Intern Med 1994; 154(20): 2311-8.
[http://dx.doi.org/10.1001/archinte.1994.00420200061007] [PMID: 7944853]

[7] Johnston SC, Pfeifer MP, McNutt R. The discussion about advance directives. Patient and physician opinions regarding when and how it should be conducted. Arch Intern Med 1995; 155(10): 1025-30.
[http://dx.doi.org/10.1001/archinte.1995.00430100047005] [PMID: 7748044]

[8] Pfeifer MP, Sidorov JE, Smith AC, Boero JF, Evans AT, Settle MB. The discussion of end-of-life medical care by primary care patients and physicians: a multicenter study using structured qualitative interviews. J Gen Intern Med 1994; 9(2): 82-8.
[http://dx.doi.org/10.1007/BF02600206] [PMID: 8164082]

[9] Seymour J, Gott M, Bellamy G, Ahmedzai SH, Clark D. Planning for the end of life: the views of older people about advance care statements. Soc Sci Med 2004; 59(1): 57-68.
[http://dx.doi.org/10.1016/j.socscimed.2003.10.005] [PMID: 15087143]

[10] Carrese JA, Mullaney JL, Faden RR, Finucane TE. Planning for death but not serious future illness: qualitative study of housebound elderly patients. BMJ 2002; 325(7356): 125.
[http://dx.doi.org/10.1136/bmj.325.7356.125] [PMID: 12130597]

[11] Samsi K, Manthorpe J. 'I live for today': a qualitative study investigating older people's attitudes to advance planning. Health Soc Care Community 2011; 19(1): 52-9.
[http://dx.doi.org/10.1111/j.1365-2524.2010.00948.x] [PMID: 20846274]

[12] Gamble ER, McDonald PJ, Lichstein PR. Knowledge, attitudes, and behavior of elderly persons regarding living wills. Arch Intern Med 1991; 151(2): 277-80.
[http://dx.doi.org/10.1001/archinte.1991.00400020049011] [PMID: 1992955]

[13] Winland-Brown JE. Death, denial, and defeat: older patients and advance directives. Adv Pract Nurs Q 1998; 4(2): 36-40.
[PMID: 9874949]

[14] Bradley EH, Peiris V, Wetle T. Discussions about end-of-life care in nursing homes. J Am Geriatr Soc 1998; 46(10): 1235-41.
[http://dx.doi.org/10.1111/j.1532-5415.1998.tb04539.x] [PMID: 9777905]

[15] Gordon NP, Shade SB. Advance directives are more likely among seniors asked about end-of-life care preferences. Arch Intern Med 1999; 159(7): 701-4.
[http://dx.doi.org/10.1001/archinte.159.7.701] [PMID: 10218749]

[16] McCarthy EP, Pencina MJ, Kelly-Hayes M, *et al.* Advance care planning and health care preferences of community-dwelling elders: the Framingham Heart Study. J Gerontol A Biol Sci Med Sci 2008; 63(9): 951-9.
[http://dx.doi.org/10.1093/gerona/63.9.951] [PMID: 18840800]

[17] Li JY, Yong TY, McNeill D, *et al.* Prevalence of resuscitation orders among residents from aged care facilities admitted to general medical units. Geriatr Gerontol Int 2012; 12(2): 364.
[http://dx.doi.org/10.1111/j.1447-0594.2011.00774.x] [PMID: 22449063]

[18] Markson L, Clark J, Glantz L, Lamberton V, Kern D, Stollerman G. The doctor's role in discussing advance preferences for end-of-life care: perceptions of physicians practicing in the VA. J Am Geriatr Soc 1997; 45(4): 399-406.
[http://dx.doi.org/10.1111/j.1532-5415.1997.tb05162.x] [PMID: 9100706]

[19] Schonfeld TL, Stevens EA, Lampman MA, Lyons WL. Assessing challenges in end-of-life conversations with elderly patients with multiple morbidities. Am J Hosp Palliat Care 2012; 29(4): 260-7.
[http://dx.doi.org/10.1177/1049909111418778] [PMID: 21868427]

[20] Stewart F, Goddard C, Schiff R, Hall S. Advanced care planning in care homes for older people: a qualitative study of the views of care staff and families. Age Ageing 2011; 40(3): 330-5.
[http://dx.doi.org/10.1093/ageing/afr006] [PMID: 21345840]

[21] Clarke A, Seymour J. "At the foot of a very long ladder": discussing the end of life with older people and informal caregivers. J Pain Symptom Manage 2010; 40(6): 857-69.
[http://dx.doi.org/10.1016/j.jpainsymman.2010.02.027] [PMID: 20813494]

[22] Froggatt K, Vaughan S, Bernard C, Wild D. Advance care planning in care homes for older people: an English perspective. Palliat Med 2009; 23(4): 332-8.
[http://dx.doi.org/10.1177/0269216309103802] [PMID: 19324923]

[23] Steinhauser KE, Clipp EC, McNeilly M, Christakis NA, McIntyre LM, Tulsky JA. In search of a good

death: observations of patients, families, and providers. Ann Intern Med 2000; 132(10): 825-32. [http://dx.doi.org/10.7326/0003-4819-132-10-200005160-00011] [PMID: 10819707]

[24] Scott IA, Mitchell GK, Reymond EJ, Daly MP. Difficult but necessary conversations--the case for advance care planning. Med J Aust 2013; 199(10): 662-6. [http://dx.doi.org/10.5694/mja13.10158] [PMID: 24237095]

[25] Houben CH, Spruit MA, Groenen MT, Wouters EF, Janssen DJ. Efficacy of advance care planning: a systematic review and meta-analysis. J Am Med Dir Assoc 2014; 15(7): 477-89. [http://dx.doi.org/10.1016/j.jamda.2014.01.008] [PMID: 24598477]

[26] Baker A, Leak P, Ritchie LD, Lee AJ, Fielding S. Anticipatory care planning and integration: a primary care pilot study aimed at reducing unplanned hospitalisation. Br J Gen Pract 2012; 62(595): e113-20. [http://dx.doi.org/10.3399/bjgp12X625175] [PMID: 22520788]

[27] Heyland DK, Dodek P, Rocker G, *et al.* What matters most in end-of-life care: perceptions of seriously ill patients and their family members. CMAJ 2006; 174(5): 627-33. [http://dx.doi.org/10.1503/cmaj.050626] [PMID: 16505458]

[28] Kapo J, Morrison LJ, Liao S. Palliative care for the older adult. J Palliat Med 2007; 10(1): 185-209. [http://dx.doi.org/10.1089/jpm.2006.9989] [PMID: 17298269]

[29] Walke LM, Gallo WT, Tinetti ME, Fried TR. The burden of symptoms among community-dwelling older persons with advanced chronic disease. Arch Intern Med 2004; 164(21): 2321-4. [http://dx.doi.org/10.1001/archinte.164.21.2321] [PMID: 15557410]

[30] Bruera E, Kuehn N, Miller MJ, Selmser P, Macmillan K. The Edmonton Symptom Assessment System (ESAS): a simple method for the assessment of palliative care patients. J Palliat Care 1991; 7(2): 6-9. [PMID: 1714502]

[31] Portenoy RK, Thaler HT, Kornblith AB, *et al.* The Memorial Symptom Assessment Scale: an instrument for the evaluation of symptom prevalence, characteristics and distress. Eur J Cancer 1994; 30A(9): 1326-36. [http://dx.doi.org/10.1016/0959-8049(94)90182-1] [PMID: 7999421]

[32] de Haes JC, van Knippenberg FC, Neijt JP. Measuring psychological and physical distress in cancer patients: structure and application of the Rotterdam Symptom Checklist. Br J Cancer 1990; 62(6): 1034-8. [http://dx.doi.org/10.1038/bjc.1990.434] [PMID: 2257209]

[33] Pautex S, Michon A, Guedira M, *et al.* Pain in severe dementia: self-assessment or observational scales? J Am Geriatr Soc 2006; 54(7): 1040-5. [http://dx.doi.org/10.1111/j.1532-5415.2006.00766.x] [PMID: 16866673]

[34] Holmes HM, Hayley DC, Alexander GC, Sachs GA. Reconsidering medication appropriateness for patients late in life. Arch Intern Med 2006; 166(6): 605-9. [http://dx.doi.org/10.1001/archinte.166.6.605] [PMID: 16567597]

Closing Remarks: Chronic Diseases In Geriatric Medicine

The prevalence of chronic diseases in the older population aged ≥65 years has generally increased over time [1, 2]. One of the key questions is whether an increase in life expectancy is accompanied by a concurrent postponement of functional limitations and disability. One of the challenges in older people is the need to manage multiple coexisting chronic diseases.

Multiple coexisting chronic diseases in an individual increase sharply with age, affecting about two-thirds of people aged 65 years and older [3 - 5]. Older patients with multiple chronic diseases experience lower quality of life, disability, dependence and increased hospital admissions [3, 6, 7]. As a result care coordination is essential to meet challenges arising from older people with multiple chronic diseases. Rigid application of clinical practice guidelines intended for single disorders should also be avoided to minimise adverse drug reaction, polypharmacy and unnecessary cost [8].

In older people, comprehensive geriatric assessment provides an important structured framework within which clinicians can integrate holistic assessment and treatment in the presence of complex comorbidities [9]. This is particularly important among frail older people who often also have multiple complex chronic conditions. Frailty often coexists with many chronic disorders because of common risk factors or underlying pathophysiologies, or because one disorder is a complication of another, or its treatment [10].

To meet the needs of older people with chronic diseases, social and economic inequalities in access to health care have to be eliminated. To achieve these needs, age discrimination should be countered and the challenges posed by multiple chronic diseases addressed. As discussed in this book, age discrimination is apparent in primary and secondary prevention of cardiovascular disease and treatment of stroke [11 - 13]. In cancer care among older people, fewer diagnostic and staging procedures are done and less evidence-based treatment is given to older people, even after taking frailty into account [14]. Even for drugs frequently prescribed in older age, older people tend to be excluded from clinical trials that would generate evidence to inform their treatment [15]. These barriers need to be overcome to better meet the needs of older people with chronic illnesses.

A substantial proportion of morbidity and mortality due to chronic diseases occurs in older people. Primary prevention in adults younger than 60 years will improve health in their older age, but much of the potential to reduce disease burden will come from effective primary, secondary and tertiary prevention targeting the older population. Although population ageing

Tuck Yean Yong (Ed)

is driving the worldwide epidemic of chronic diseases, substantial untapped potential exists to modify the relation between chronological age and health.

REFERENCES

[1] Freedman VA, Martin LG. Contribution of chronic conditions to aggregate changes in old-age functioning. Am J Public Health 2000; 90(11): 1755-60.
[http://dx.doi.org/10.2105/AJPH.90.11.1755] [PMID: 11076245]

[2] Meinow B, Parker M, Kåreholt I, Thorslund M. Complex health problems in the oldest old in Sweden 1992–2002. Eur J Ageing 2006; 3: 98-106.
[http://dx.doi.org/10.1007/s10433-006-0027-z]

[3] Wolff JL, Starfield B, Anderson G. Prevalence, expenditures, and complications of multiple chronic conditions in the elderly. Arch Intern Med 2002; 162(20): 2269-76.
[http://dx.doi.org/10.1001/archinte.162.20.2269] [PMID: 12418941]

[4] Caughey GE, Ramsay EN, Vitry AI, *et al.* Comorbid chronic diseases, discordant impact on mortality in older people: a 14-year longitudinal population study. J Epidemiol Community Health 2010; 64(12): 1036-42.
[http://dx.doi.org/10.1136/jech.2009.088260] [PMID: 19854745]

[5] Kirchberger I, Meisinger C, Heier M, *et al.* Patterns of multimorbidity in the aged population. Results from the KORA-Age study. PLoS One 2012; 7(1): e30556.
[http://dx.doi.org/10.1371/journal.pone.0030556] [PMID: 22291986]

[6] Fortin M, Bravo G, Hudon C, *et al.* Relationship between multimorbidity and health-related quality of life of patients in primary care. Qual Life Res 2006; 15(1): 83-91.
[http://dx.doi.org/10.1007/s11136-005-8661-z] [PMID: 16411033]

[7] Wolff JL, Boult C, Boyd C, Anderson G. Newly reported chronic conditions and onset of functional dependency. J Am Geriatr Soc 2005; 53(5): 851-5.
[http://dx.doi.org/10.1111/j.1532-5415.2005.53262.x] [PMID: 15877563]

[8] Boyd CM, Darer J, Boult C, Fried LP, Boult L, Wu AW. Clinical practice guidelines and quality of care for older patients with multiple comorbid diseases: implications for pay for performance. JAMA 2005; 294(6): 716-24.
[http://dx.doi.org/10.1001/jama.294.6.716] [PMID: 16091574]

[9] Stuck AE, Siu AL, Wieland GD, Adams J, Rubenstein LZ. Comprehensive geriatric assessment: a meta-analysis of controlled trials. Lancet 1993; 342(8878): 1032-6.
[http://dx.doi.org/10.1016/0140-6736(93)92884-V] [PMID: 8105269]

[10] van Weel C, Schellevis FG. Comorbidity and guidelines: conflicting interests. Lancet 2006; 367(9510): 550-1.
[http://dx.doi.org/10.1016/S0140-6736(06)68198-1] [PMID: 16488782]

[11] Ramsay SE, Morris RW, Papacosta O, Lennon LT, Thomas MC, Whincup PH. Secondary prevention of coronary heart disease in older British men: extent of inequalities before and after implementation of the National Service Framework. J Public Health (Oxf) 2005; 27(4): 338-43.
[http://dx.doi.org/10.1093/pubmed/fdi053] [PMID: 16162637]

[12] Ramsay SE, Whincup PH, Wannamethee SG, *et al.* Missed opportunities for secondary prevention of cerebrovascular disease in elderly British men from 1999 to 2005: a population-based study. J Public Health (Oxf) 2007; 29(3): 251-7. [http://dx.doi.org/10.1093/pubmed/fdm040] [PMID: 17584949]

[13] Luker JA, Wall K, Bernhardt J, Edwards I, Grimmer-Somers KA. Patients' age as a determinant of care received following acute stroke: a systematic review. BMC Health Serv Res 2011; 11: 161. [http://dx.doi.org/10.1186/1472-6963-11-161] [PMID: 21729329]

[14] Turner NJ, Haward RA, Mulley GP, Selby PJ. Cancer in old age--is it inadequately investigated and treated? BMJ 1999; 319(7205): 309-12. [http://dx.doi.org/10.1136/bmj.319.7205.309] [PMID: 10426753]

[15] Konrat C, Boutron I, Trinquart L, Auleley GR, Ricordeau P, Ravaud P. Underrepresentation of elderly people in randomised controlled trials. The example of trials of 4 widely prescribed drugs. PLoS One 2012; 7(3): e33559. [http://dx.doi.org/10.1371/journal.pone.0033559] [PMID: 22479411]

SUBJECT INDEX

Q

R

S

T

V

Made in the USA
Las Vegas, NV
04 November 2026

57431559R00131